SCHIZOPHRENIA: THE FACTS
(second edition) Ming T. Tsuang
and Stephen V. Faraone

THYROID DISEASE:
THE FACTS
(third edition) R. I. S. Bayliss and
W. M. G. Tunbridge

TOURETTE SYNDROME:
THE FACTS
(second edition) Mary Robertson
and Simon Baron-Cohen

OXFORD MEDICAL PUBLICATIONS

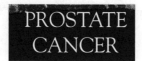

PROSTATE
CANCER

the**facts**

the**facts**
ALSO AVAILABLE IN THE SERIES

PROSTATE CANCER

the**facts**

Malcolm Mason
Section of Oncology and Palliative Medicine
University of Wales
College of Medicine
Wales

and

Leslie Moffat
Consultant in Urology
Aberdeen Royal Infirmary
Scotland

OXFORD
UNIVERSITY PRESS

OXFORD
UNIVERSITY PRESS

Great Clarendon Street, Oxford OX2 6DP

Oxford University Press is a department of the University of Oxford.
It furthers the University's objective of excellence in research,
scholarship, and education by publishing worldwide in

Oxford New York
Auckland Bangkok Buenos Aires Cape Town Chennai
Dar es Salaam Delhi Hong Kong Istanbul Karachi Kolkata
Kuala Lumpur Madrid Melbourne Mexico City Mumbai Nairobi
São Paulo Shanghai Taipei Tokyo Toronto

Oxford is a registered trade mark of Oxford University Press
in the UK and in certain other countries

Published in the United States
by Oxford University Press Inc., New York

A catalogue record for this title is available from the British Library

Library of Congress Cataloging in Publication Data
(Data available)

ISBN 0 19 263144 6 (Pbk)

10 9 8 7 6 5 4 3 2 1

Typeset by Integra Software Services Pvt. Ltd, Pondicherry, India
www.integra-india.com
Printed in Great Britain
on acid-free paper by
TJ International Ltd, Padstow, Cornwall

the**facts**

CONTENTS

Preface

Prostate cancer has become one of the commonest male cancers in the Western world. There is a plethora of information about the disease, especially on the Internet. In some instances, there is a 'spin' or 'hype' imparted to the information that is unhelpful or even may be unethical. In this book, we have, as two practising doctors, one an oncologist and the other a surgeon, tried to give the information about this complex disease as it really is, without bias.

This is a book for those patients and their carers who wish to go beyond the patient leaflets that are now, fortunately, readily available. Medical information can be impenetrable at worst or inaccessible at best. More detailed explanations of certain aspects are given here, in the hope that the interested layperson can begin to penetrate medical thinking, be guided through a morass of data, and to allow them to arrive at an informed position. Some degree of repetition is inevitable in this book—patients with prostate cancer vary so much that not all chapters will be relevant to all patients, and those dipping into different, selected chapters will, hopefully find the information that they need without too much cross-referencing.

We hope that, through this book, we can in some small way help society as a whole to take stock of the dilemma that is prostate cancer.

Malcolm Mason
Leslie Moffat

2003

1
Introduction

The prostate – what is it, where is it, and how is it assessed?

The prostate is a gland, just below the bladder in men (Fig. 1.1). It is not found in women. It should be noted that the word is 'prostate' and not 'prostrate' – its function is imperfectly understood, but seems to be entirely linked to human reproduction. It produces substances that are used to nourish the sperm in semen, and which affect the degree of viscosity of the semen (turning it into a jelly and then later on back into a fluid). It is the best source of hormones called 'prostaglandins', which were first isolated from prostatic tissue. Prostatic secretions may also have an effect on the female reproductive tract.

The seminal vesicles lie alongside the prostate and look like small bunches of grapes. They produce over half the volume of the ejaculate, producing substances such as sugars that nourish the sperm and activate them prior to ejaculation. They drain into the lower area of the prostate. They are usually removed by the operation termed a radical prostatectomy, and irradiated if necessary during treatment by radical radiotherapy.

The vas deferens is a tube that joins the testicles to the interior of the prostate. The sperm are released through the ejaculatory duct in the centre of the urethra, which travels through the centre of the prostate. There is a vas on both sides to drain both testicles.

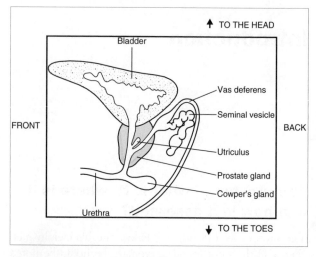

Figure 1.1 Cross-sectional diagram of the prostate gland, indicating the surrounding structures.

The nerves that control erection of the penis lie at the sides of the prostate. These nerves can be damaged during treatment for prostate cancer, resulting in impotence.

During embryonic development, the prostate wraps itself around the urethra, the tube draining the bladder. It therefore becomes obvious that if the prostate gland enlarges, it can cause obstruction to the flow of urine.

Almost all men have a degree of enlargement of the prostate, which is called 'benign prostatic hyperplasia' (BPH). BPH starts in middle age or even earlier, for reasons that are still not understood, but the male hormone testosterone is implicated as such enlargement would not occur if a male is castrated before the age of 12.

In a young man of 16, the prostate is slightly bigger than a small walnut. In a man of 80 it can be as large as an orange. Although the prostate is situated deep within the pelvis, it is fortuitous that the back portion of the prostate can be felt through the rectum (the 'back passage') and this is the basis for the examination whereby a doctor or nurse places his or her gloved finger in the rectum. Two things about the prostate can be assessed by this examination: first, the size of the prostate, and second, the consistency of the prostate, which can sometimes indicate cancer of the prostate.

Cancer of the prostate feels very hard. Occasionally a small nodule can be felt on the prostate and this can be displayed by taking an image called a 'transrectal ultrasound' (TRUS). TRUS also takes advantage of the proximity of the prostate and the rectum. A TRUS probe is inserted into the rectum and takes the place of the doctor's finger. Using ultrasonic waves, a picture can be produced on a screen and may indicate the presence of a cancer and/or guide a needle used to take biopsy samples of the prostate. This is discussed in more detail elsewhere, but a hypoechoic area (meaning that the area does not produce an echo with the same intensity as the remainder of the prostate) is often associated with malignancy.

Usually, if a TRUS is done, biopsies will be taken. This is done by inserting a needle through the probe, usually taking six to eight samples but sometimes more. A biopsy will only be taken after antibiotics have been given either by injection or as tablets and further antibiotics may be given later, after the biopsy. An expert pathologist can determine, from the biopsy sample of the prostate, whether or not cancer is present, and, if it is, the *grade* of the cancer. This is an important feature which is discussed in another chapter.

The body is composed of many billions of cells organized into tissues and organs. Nature has decreed that animals, including man, develop and maintain their structure by allowing cells the ability to divide and grow, to replace cells that die after injury or after a cell has reached its allotted life span. It is a miracle that so few of these cells go off the track. Most behave and live ordinary lives, growing, dividing and then dying when appropriate. Every day, in the human body, millions of such cell divisions are taking place. An essential part of this process is the replication of a cell's entire DNA content – the genetic 'blueprint' for human life. This process is akin to copying the contents of a huge computer 'hard disk' but is vastly more complicated and is not error-free. It is estimated that, just as computers make mistakes when files are copied, every day in every person several thousand 'mistakes' are made during cell division. The miracle is that, every day, each of these mistakes is detected and dealt with; just occasionally, one slips through the net.

Occasionally, such a mistake, if uncorrected, allows cells to start developing abnormally and find a way of bypassing normal control mechanisms. This allows the number of cells in a particular area to grow in an uncontrolled way that could lead to cancer. Nearly all cancers start as a series of mistakes, and arise from just one cell. However, most 'mistakes' will have no effect, or, at worst, lead to a benign growth that is not a cancer.

Benign (non-cancerous) enlargement of the prostate (also called 'benign prostatic hyperplasia')

Not all 'growths' arise because of mistakes during DNA replication at cell division. Some result from a change in the normal balance of factors – including hormones such as testosterone – that encourage the healthy growth of an organ such as the prostate. This occurs in other hormone-responsive organs, including the breast in women with oestrogen.

Benign enlargement of the prostate with age has already been referred to. Under the microscope it can be seen that the vast majority of this enlargement is due to an increase in the number of cells. This is called 'benign prostatic hyperplasia' (BPH). Despite the increase in the number of cells, this condition is entirely benign or non-malignant.

Malignancy or cancer – which is it?

Malignancy and cancer mean the same thing. As discussed, in hyperplasia the number of cells increases. Despite this, there is still a degree of order in the increased number of cells and although the prostate may continue to grow, its cells show no signs of leaving their companion cells or attempting to go elsewhere by invading any other areas of the body.

In malignancy, two processes occur.

Invasion

The first process is *invasion*. Cells, which have become malignant, start to invade into the area outside their normal territory. They can invade into blood vessels, but in the prostate, they also particularly tend to invade along the channels of the nerves in the prostate. Such cells are able to move outside the capsule of the prostate, resulting in local advancement of cancer.

Metastasis

The other hallmark of malignancy is the capacity of the malignant cells which have left outside their normal position to set up colonies in more remote parts of the body. This is *metastasis* – the formation of 'secondaries'. These colonies continue to grow in size and number, beginning to damage normal cells in areas to where they have spread.

In prostate cancer, metastases spread to lymph nodes and elsewhere, but have a peculiar propensity to settle in bone. Why this is so is a mystery, but it signifies a complex relationship between prostate cancer cells and bone cells, that encourages such a pattern of spread. Bone metastases can be identified by plain radiographs or bone scans.

Table 1.1 Age-standardized incidence rates per 100 000 for cancer of the prostate

Country	Incidence
US: black	137.0
US, Hawaii: white	108.2
US: white	100.8
Canada	64.7
US, Hawaii: Japanese	64.2
US, Hawaii, Chinese	62.9
Zimbabwe, Harare: European	55.7
Sweden	55.3
US, Puerto Rico	54.7
South Australia	53.6
Austria, Tyrol	51.6
France, Calvados	50.5
US, Hawaii: Filipino	49.5
US, Hawaii: Hawaiian	42.1
Finland	41.3
The Netherlands	39.6
Germany: Saarland	35.9
Brazil, Goiania	35.2
Uruguay, Montevideo	32.6
UK, Scotland	31.2
Denmark	31.0
Ireland, Southern	30.9
Zimbabwe, Harare: African	29.2
UK, England and Wales	28.0
Italy, Genoa	24.7
Czech Republic	24.1
Israel: all Jews	23.9
Germany: eastern states	23.7
Ecuador, Quito	22.4
Spain, Zaragoza	19.7
Peru, Lima	19.4
Kuwait: non-Kuwaitis	18.3
Philippines, Manila	17.6
Argentina, Concordia	16.2
Poland, Warsaw City	15.7
Yugoslavia, Vojvodina	14.7
Japan, Hiroshima	10.9
Israel: non-Jews	10.4
Singapore: Chinese	9.8
Hong Kong	7.9

India, Bombay	7.9
Kuwait: Kuwaitis	6.5
China, Shanghai	2.3
Viet Nam: Hanoi	1.2
Korea, Kangwa	0.9

Geographical aspects of prostate cancer

Prostate cancer is common in all Western countries and is particularly common in the USA (Table 1.1). It is particularly common in the black population of North America, where the disease tends to present about 10 years earlier than it would in North American whites. The reason for this unfortunate fact is as yet obscure, but is probably related to a genetic component.

The causes of prostate cancer

There are a number of risk factors. Ageing (particularly over 70 years) is thought to be the strongest risk factor and there is no doubt that as a population becomes more elderly the incidence rates of prostate cancer also increase in that population.

This contributes to an impression that prostate cancer is becoming more common, an impression which may be exaggerated by the ageing population. Age *per se* is not a cause of prostate cancer. It is simply that, the longer a man lives, the more chance his prostate's cells have of going awry.

Diet

The more animal fats that are consumed by a nation, the greater the risk of prostate cancer in its men. Vegetarians are said to be at much smaller risk of developing prostate cancer, perhaps by as much as 50 per cent. The body's fat content affects the handling of testosterone and this may be the link between fat and prostate cancer.

Chinese and Japanese men have a much lower rate of prostate cancer than North Americans and Europeans. There is also an interesting observation that Japanese men, who have moved from Japan to North America, increase their risk of prostate cancer towards that of the local population.

It is difficult to disentangle the effects of diet of genetic make-up. Prostate cancer is more common in countries where the risk of heart disease is higher, but both could be due to a mixture of dietary and genetic effects.

Possible protective factors in diet

Antioxidants Oxygen is ubiquitous in the human body. The laws of chemistry result in a tendency for complex biological molecules to have oxygen added to them – a process called 'oxidation'. Paradoxically, and despite the fact that oxygen is essential to fuel human life, oxidation causes damage to complex biological materials, including DNA, and may be one factor that causes cancer. A number of substances found in food can counteract this happening. They are therefore called 'antioxidants'. Examples of antioxidants are found in Table 1.2.

Lycopenes, which are found in cooked tomatoes, may have a mild protective effect but this remains to be proved beyond all reasonable doubt.

Table 1.2 Antioxidants – some examples

Vitamin E (the most important natural antioxidant, acts with selenium)
• Found in margarine

Vitamin A (Beta-carotene)
• Found in carrots

Vitamin C
• Found in fresh fruit and vegetables

Various diets have been devised, and the effect of adding compounds such as retinoids, carotenoids, and vitamin C to an adequate diet continues to be discussed.

Selenium, which is an essential trace element found in plants, enters the food chain by plant ingestion and is essentially dependent on soil concentration. Selenium may protect against the action of certain carcinogens.

Soya products are said to inhibit prostate cancer. The compounds thought to be responsible are called 'isoflavonoids'.

Industrial exposure

Exposure to cadmium, which can occur in men working in copper smelting, seems to increase the risk of prostate cancer. Some authors have claimed that exposure to ultra-violet light increases the risk of prostate cancer, but this is far from proven. In general, though, it is unlikely that industrial or occupational exposure is responsible for the vast majority of prostate cancers.

Sexual behaviour

There have been a number of studies to investigate whether the younger that a man becomes sexually active, the more he will increase his risk of prostate cancer. The hypothesis is that such men will have had multiple partners and may have been exposed to more viruses than others. However, there is no firm evidence linking sexually acquired viruses with prostate cancer and on current evidence there is nothing that one can do to modify sexual lifestyle, to reduce the risk of prostate cancer.

2 Assessment of the severity and extent of prostate cancer

Describing the extent of prostate cancer

The process of defining the extent of a cancer is called 'staging'. The most widely used system to classify the spread of prostate cancer is the TNM staging system. This stands for tumour, nodes, and metastases.

T-stage – the primary tumour

The T-stage indicates the degree to which the tumour has grown in the prostate itself. The tumour is assigned a stage ranging from T1 to T4, defined as follows:

T1   Tumour not palpable or visible

T1a   Tumour present in <5% of tissue resected at TURP infiltrated by cancer

T1b   >5% of tissue resected at TURP infiltrated by cancer

T1c   Tumour found on needle biopsy only

T2   A tumour that can be felt by the physician, but is confined within prostate

T2a   One side involved

T2b   Both sides involved

T3   Spread of tumour through the prostatic capsule

T3a   To surrounding tissues

T3b   To the seminal vesicle(s)

T4   Tumour is fixed or invades adjacent structures: bladder neck, external sphincter, rectum, levator muscles, pelvic wall

Nodes

This refers to lymph nodes. We have seen how tumours invade along the nerves of the prostate and once outside the capsule, tumour cells go into the lymphatic system. There are concentrations of lymphatic tissue called 'lymph nodes' along the channels. These may be likened to sentry points along the highway. Bacterial cells are dealt with in the lymph nodes and sometimes the tumour can similarly be successfully destroyed by the immune system. However, tumours can also grow in the nodes and this is assessed in the following way:

N0   No regional lymph node metastasis

N1   Metastasis in single regional lymph node, <2 cm in largest dimension

N2   Metastasis in single regional lymph node, >2 cm but <5 cm in largest dimension

N3   Metastasis in regional lymph node >5 cm in largest dimension.

It is possible to remove these lymph nodes surgically and this may be done as part of a wider operation; in some cases this might cure the patient.

Metastasis

This represents spread of cancer outside the normal areas of the prostate, or the nearest (regional) lymph nodes to a remote point. This particularly occurs in bones, but the cancer can spread to other organs, such as the liver or to lymph nodes that are not in the vicinity of the prostate, e.g. the neck. Metastasis can be grouped as follows:

M0   No distant metastasis

M1   Distant metastasis

M1a Metastasis in non-regional lymph nodes

M1b Metastasis in bone

M1c Metastasis at other site.

How do images show how advanced a prostate cancer is?

TRUS

The first investigation is likely to be a transrectal ultrasound scan (TRUS). This involves the patient lying on his side and the radiologist or surgeon inserting a probe into his rectum. This uses ultrasound, high-frequency sound waves, to obtain a picture of the prostate. The doctor will be looking for areas that do not have normal but reduced echoes (hypoechoic areas) Using a spring-loaded gun, a needle can be fired into the prostate and biopsies taken. These may be restricted to an abnormal area but often three biopsies are taken from both lobes of the prostate – six biopsies or more in all. This may be uncomfortable but is not as painful as one might expect. The biopsies are then sent for examination at the pathology laboratory.

In early cancer, the patient's doctor may request CAT (computed axial tomography) or an MRI (magnetic resonance imaging) scans.

CAT scan

This is a special type of x-ray where pictures are taken in many different directions and a computer then works out a final picture.

MRI scan

This uses magnetic rays rather than x-rays and is believed to be in some situations more accurate.

Other methods

The presence of spread outside the lymph nodes or the prostate is found in two main ways. Prostate cancer seems to spread preferentially to the bones, particularly the spine and pelvis. These secondaries show up as denser areas on x-ray pictures and an ordinary x-ray is a good way of showing up this type of disease.

An additional method is a bone scan. This is carried out by injecting a radioactive isotope, which goes specially to the bones, and can be shown up by scanning all the bones after a short period of time. The radioactivity does not last long and it is perfectly safe to mix with people in company after 2 days.

How do we measure how aggressive a prostate cancer is?

When a biopsy is taken a pathologist looks at the tissue. He or she is skilled in looking at tissue under a microscope and analysing and diagnosing and *grading* a tumour. One measurement that can be made is the degree of aggression of the tumour. One scheme, which has proved useful, was first described by Gleason. He looked at the patterns of growth of malignant tissue and graded them from fairly inactive to very active (Table 2.1). He looked at the most predominant pattern and then at the next most predominant pattern and added

Table 2.1 Gleason's guide to tumour aggression

Cancerous tissue pattern	Gleason grade
Non-aggressive tumour	
Closely packed, well-defined glands within the prostate	1
Less uniformly shaped glands	2
Irregular glands of variable size	3
A mass of fused glands	4
Aggressive tumour	
Few, or no, visible glands; very little difference between them	5

the two grades together to obtain a score, e.g. Gleason $3 + 2 = 5$.

The final figure is a sum score and is known to relate to survival – the higher the number the shorter the survival. On its own, this may not give the whole story, but it may help a patient to decide whether to have aggressive treatment.

PSA

PSA stands for 'prostate-specific antigen'. This is a protein that is detected in the bloodstream of almost all adult men. The protein has a role in adjusting the stickiness of semen.

As men age, their prostates become bigger. This tends to make the level of PSA rise. In addition, more of the PSA 'leaks' into the bloodstream as men get older. PSA measures activity in prostate tissue. It has been found that various conditions are associated with an increase of PSA above normal levels (Table 2.2). PSA increases with age,

Table 2.2 Conditions associated with change in PSA

Result	Condition or activity causing change in PSA
Rise	Prostate cancer
Rise	Benign prostatic hyperplasia
Rise	Prostate biopsy
Rise	Prostatitis (usually caused by infection)
Rise	Prostate manipulation (i.e. DRE or TRUS)
Rise	Cycling!
Decrease	Hormone therapy
Decrease	Prostatectomy (removal of prostate)
Variable	Sex
Variable	Exercise

DRE, digital rectal examination; TRUS, transrectal ultrasound.

and normal levels have been calculated for each age group. Patients with prostate cancer usually have an increase in PSA.

The PSA level can be a useful method of determining response to treatment, whether after surgery to remove the prostate (radical prostatectomy), after radiotherapy, or after hormonal treatment in more advanced cancers.

Prostate cancer symptoms

There are generally no symptoms associated with early prostate cancer. However, if and when they appear, the symptoms of prostate cancer and BPH are very similar. These tend to involve problems with 'the waterworks'. Patients often experience:

- difficulty or pain when passing urine;
- the need to pass urine more often (frequency);
- broken sleep due to increased visits to pass urine;
- waiting for long periods before the urine flows (hesitancy);
- the feeling that the bladder has not emptied fully.

These symptoms are sometimes associated with early disease and can be the first signs of prostate enlargement. Other symptoms, which can be associated with later stage disease, are:

- blood in the urine (unusual);
- pain in the pelvis or loins;
- blood in the sperm (very rare);
- general bone pain;
- weight loss.

All these symptoms should be reported to your doctor so that they can be investigated, although they may be caused by something other than prostate cancer.

Questions to ask the doctor

General

- Do you think that I may have a problem with my prostate?
- What tests should I consider and what is involved?
- If you find prostate cancer, what is the next step?

After receipt of the test results

- My PSA blood test result is raised. How high is the result and what could this mean?
- How certain can you be that I have prostate cancer and not another prostate condition?
- What can you tell me about the cancer (size, position, speed, and growth)?
- Which do you feel would be the most suitable treatment for me and why?
- If I choose to be treated, will the treatment relieve my symptoms?
- What are the side-effects of the treatment and how might they affect my lifestyle?

3

Risks and benefits of screening and radical treatment – a guide

Almost any lifestyle has associated risks. It is not perhaps surprising that parachuting in the USA carries a risk of 19 000 times that of playing Association Football in England and Wales. Climbing in England and Wales carries 130 times the risk of playing football. Surgical anaesthesia in England in 1986 had a risk of death of 5.4 cases per million operations.

One of the most difficult aspects of prostate cancer is that the decision-making process is presented to patients as a 'risks versus benefits' equation. This is a difficult concept, particularly when many of the risks seem abstract at a time when patients may have no symptoms whatsoever. It is also a difficult subject for healthcare professionals to convey well, and this section is an attempt to represent some of the issues in a graphical manner.

No-one knows for certain how many prostate cancers are treated unnecessarily, or how many which needed treatment were subject to 'watchful waiting'. Neither do we know – for certain – whether current treatments cure prostate cancers. This is an important fact, which has an impact both on screening and on the selection of radical treatment or watchful waiting. We will consider screening and radical treatment in turn. The famous urologist Walt Whitmore summed up the dilemma thus:

Is a cure possible in patients in whom it might be necessary?
Is a cure necessary in patients in whom it might be possible?

It is believed that up to 80% of *all* men develop prostate cancer by the age of 80. Nothing like this number of men suffer harm from their cancer, implying, that in most men prostate cancer is a harmless illness.

This chapter considers some hypothetical prostate cancers and assigns them a hypothetical chance of causing their hosts some harm during their lifetime. It is most important to stress that any figures presented here are purely hypothetical, to illustrate the ways in which such tumours might affect risk. They should not be treated as an accurate estimate, since for most situations we simply do not know what the actual figure is. These figures should not be used by patients or by doctors for making decisions about an actual patient with the same disease characteristics as are selected here.

First, let us consider the question of screening. Let us assume to begin with that, if a small prostate cancer is present in a patient who is fit and well, it will be detected. How likely is it that it is a significant cancer? This question is impossible to answer with any accuracy, but experts believe that, overall, around one in seven of such cancers are 'significant', the other six being cancers which would not affect a patient's life if they were left untreated. This can be represented pictorially as shown in Fig. 3.1.

However, this estimate (even if it is accurate), is an overall figure, which is of limited value for an individual

   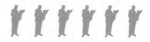

For every man who is harmed   There are another 6 who are not
by his prostrate cancer

Figure 3.1 Diagram to indicate difference between a 'harmful' prostate cancer from a 'harmless' prostate cancer. Oncologists have no way of distinguishing between a harmful and harmless prostate cancer.

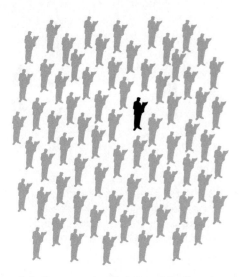

Figure 3.2 One man in 70 has a 'significant' or harmful prostate cancer, although the cancers look the same in all 70 men.

patient. To illustrate this, let us consider a patient who is found to have a small cancer, which is not visible or palpable (i.e. the prostate gland feels normal), who has a PSA in the normal range for his age, and whose Gleason sum score (see Chapter 2) is only 3. His chances of 'significant' disease might be 1 in 70 rather than 1 in 7, which would look pictorially as shown in Fig. 3.2. Even this estimate, which is also highly theoretical, takes no account of the patient's age. The younger a patient, the longer he may live, and theoretically the greater the chance his prostate cancer may have to cause him harm. For a patient aged 50, his lifetime chance of the above tumour causing him harm might be 1 in 20, whereas the same tumour, in a patient aged 80 might have a lifetime chance of causing harm of only 1 in 200.

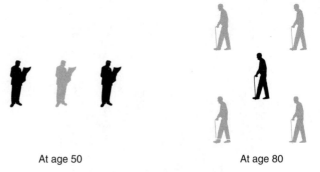

At age 50   At age 80

Figure 3.3 The risk from a cancer getting worse (disease progression) also depends on a person's age. In this example, a man with a significant prostate cancer, diagnosed at age 50, has a 2 in 3 lifetime risk of it progressing.

Now, let us consider a tumour that is palpable (can be felt on examination), but confined to the prostate gland. It has a Gleason sum score of 8. This tumour is much more likely to cause harm, at all ages, although in a younger patient it is perhaps particularly likely to have the opportunity to do so (say, at any time over the next 30 years). The risks of such a tumour – if untreated – causing harm to a man aged 50 at some stage in his lifetime might be 2 in 3. In a man aged 80, destined to live for another 5 years, it might be 1 in 5. These risks could be represented pictorially as shown in Fig. 3.3.

Note that, even in this hypothetical situation, where we have assumed that we actually know the risks (and, again, it is emphasized that we *do not*), we cannot predict with certainty what *will* happen to an individual patient, only what *might* happen. However, although the figures themselves are hypothetical, the general ranking of risk is accurate. In other words, an untreated tumour is least likely to cause harm if it is well differentiated, impalpable, associated with a low PSA, and present in an elderly man. An untreated tumour is most likely to cause harm if it is poorly differentiated, palpable, and is associated with a high PSA in a young man. Many tumours fall into the middle of these extremes – for example, a moderately differentiated tumour, which is visible on scans but not palpable, associated with a mildly elevated PSA, in a man aged 62.

All these considerations make the issues of screening and treatment more complex than it might have appeared at first sight. However, to further complicate the situation, we must return to our initial assumption – that is, that if a cancer were present, it would be detected. Unfortunately, this is not always the case. Although a combination of PSA, rectal examination, and TRUS are highly sensitive means of detecting a prostate cancer, they are far from perfect, and some patients, with significant cancers, may be wrongly labelled as being 'all clear'. Other patients, who do not have cancer, can have a scare when screening tests suggest that they do, until they are later proved to be 'all clear'.

In summary:

- Screening is not perfect. It might unnecessarily scare a man who actually does not have prostate cancer.

- Treatment is not perfect. It might cause harm to a man whose prostate cancer would not have caused him harm.

- Equally, it may well be that treatment will cure some patients, though as yet we do not have reliable evidence as to whether or not this is so.

- Treatment may prevent disease progression, which in itself could be beneficial, irrespective of whether or not it also cures people.

- Screening is not perfect. It might wrongly reassure a man who actually does have prostate cancer, but in whom it is not detected.

- If a prostate cancer is discovered, it is impossible to predict what *will* happen to the patient. It is a little easier to guess as to how likely a cancer, if untreated, *might be* to cause a man harm at some time during his lifetime, but our weighing of the risks is based on crude estimates, not facts.

- In assessing the risks to an individual, doctors would need to consider his age, the size of the tumour, its grade (Gleason sum score), and his PSA level.

This discussion is not an argument against screening or radical treatment. However, it is because of their limitations that many doctors feel that they should be evaluated in a clinical study, or clinical trial, before it is introduced. This is particularly true when the risks of radical treatment (radical prostatectomy or radical radiotherapy) are considered, and these are discussed in Chapter 4.

4
Treatment and management options

General introduction – a guide to choice of treatment

This chapter considers the different ways of treating the prostate gland. Deciding which of these options is the most appropriate can be one of the most difficult aspects of managing prostate cancer, and is often bewildering for doctor and patient alike. The reason for this difficulty is simple – *we do not know the best treatment for prostate cancer*. For a number of reasons, not the least of which may be technical, not every patient is suitable for every form of treatment. This important aspect is something that should be discussed with the specialist.

The 'success rate' after radical treatment depends on a complex and wide-ranging number of variables. It varies hugely between patients and therefore, deliberately, treatment results are not given here. Additionally, the lack of high-quality, randomized trials comparing treatments means that their respective 'success' rates are difficult to gauge.

Watchful waiting or active monitoring

Active monitoring in early disease

Watchful waiting is also known as surveillance therapy, expectant management, or observation. Some authors have now adopted the term 'active monitoring', which is probably a more accurate description of the process. Essentially, active monitoring implies that the patient has initially decided with his doctor to avoid active treatment, but to monitor the disease by estimating the PSA at several monthly intervals and tracking it.

In any other cancer, this would seem a strange concept. The reasons why active monitoring may be sensible in some patients are, first, we know that not all cancers will progress during the patient's lifetime, to cause him trouble. The other factor is that all the treatments, descriptions of which follow, have side-effects. Sometimes it is quite possible to balance up the risks of treatment, versus the risks of the disease getting worse (progressing).

We know that certain patients with early T1a cancers, diagnosed incidentally at a transurethral resection of the prostate (TURP), have between a 3 and 16 per cent chance of progressing over 8 years. If the patient has a life expectancy of less than 10 years, then active monitoring would be an option to consider seriously. Active monitoring does not imply a lack of treatment, but merely balancing the risks of treatment against the risk of complications.

Some of the early studies on active monitoring looked at patients who had a very low risk of death from cancer. Because there are no randomized control trials to show the relative survival of different treatments in different tumour stages and Gleason grades, we have to look at studies that examine the results of active monitoring in a retrospective manner; in other words, the patients are not followed forwards in time, but the numbers of patients alive or well are traced backwards from a point in time.

Gerry Chodak, a surgeon in Chicago, examined various selected series of patients with localised prostate cancer, who were treated conservatively. In the group of Gleason scores 2–4, there was a 10-year risk of 19 per cent of developing secondary disease, which increased to 40 per cent at 15 years. In the Gleason score 5–7, 42 per cent developed secondaries in 10 years and 70 per cent at 15 years. Those with Gleason scores of 8 upwards had a 74 per cent risk of developing secondary disease within 10 years and 85 per cent at 15 years.

A recent paper in the *Lancet* by Lu-Yao and Yao examined the results from the SEER database and examined the records of 60 000 patients who had had treatment or active montoring. They found that the relative survival in patients with tumours equivalent to the low Gleason scores, i.e. the 2–4 group, showed that they had an improved chance of surviving 10 years compared with a group of men of the same age. They found, however, that those equivalent to the Gleason scores 5–7 had a reduced survival, with respect to a similar group of men of the same age and that this reduction of survival was even greater in those with Gleason scores 8 and 9. There is thus limited evidence that patients with low Gleason scores can benefit from avoiding radical therapies.

Active monitoring in advanced disease

If treatments involve a major operation or potentially dangerous drugs, there is a strong argument for deferring treatment until the patient has symptoms. However, with the development of newer anti-androgens and luteinizing hormone-releasing hormone (LH-RH) analogues, the toxicity is very much less. Nonetheless, all these drug treatments carry some risk.

There are a number of other reasons why patients may wish to have earlier treatment. Some patients cannot bear the thought that their cancer is not being confronted. There is a risk that the bulk of disease increases and becomes more difficult for the tumour to be controlled. There is the very real risk that the patient may develop side-effects and spinal problems, due to a collapse of bones, with secondary disease. There is the possibility that the untreated prostate cancer may become less hormone sensitive is it develops, although the evidence for this is much less. Local progression of prostate cancer may require the patient to have an operation on his prostate, due to urinary blockage.

There is a feeling that in advanced disease, deferred treatment may reduce survival and there is also a risk that some patients could die from prostate cancer without receiving treatment if not monitored carefully.

A large trial performed by the Medical Research Council appeared to show marginally an improvement in survival, but undoubtedly a lower risk of complications. The differences were not considerable, however, and it is interesting to note that 27 patients receiving immediate treatment died from cancer of other organs, quite unrelated to their prostate cancer. The risk of death from heart disease and strokes appeared to be similar in both groups.

Watchful waiting after failure of primary therapy

Unfortunately, after a radical prostatectomy, a number of patients may find that they have what is called 'margin-positive disease'. Although this is disappointing, 50 per cent of these patients do not appear to progress and so there is an argument for managing this situation by active monitoring. It is wise to be guided by the surgeon about this.

Occasionally patients will fail after radiotherapy (external beam or brachytherapy). The levels of PSA may be very low initially and the radiotherapist will wish to look at the doubling time of the PSA, as well as the absolute levels.

In terms of active monitoring, it is important to remember that it is unfortunate if a patient has treatment, with a lot of side-effects, without benefit. Many patients who 'fail' their first treatment will still never die of their prostate cancer.

Radiotherapy

Introduction

Radical radiotherapy is reserved for men whose disease it appears possible to eradicate completely, in the hope that this will cure the patient. Radiotherapy (or x-ray therapy) is a treatment which uses high-energy x-rays to kill cancer cells. It has been known for a long time that x-rays damage cells – both normal cells and cancer cells. However, cancer cells have a reduced ability to repair x-ray-induced damage, and this is the basis for radiotherapy. Treatment is given in such a way that normal cells are able to recover, whereas cancer cells are not. There are two general methods for delivering radiotherapy:

- external beam radiotherapy, in which the patient lies on a couch, and x-rays are shone from a machine onto the pelvis, targeted at the prostate gland;
- brachytherapy, in which radioactive seeds, which give out x-rays, are implanted into the prostate gland, usually under a general anaesthetic and in the operating theatre.

These are considered here in turn.

External beam radiotherapy

This is the most common form of radiotherapy. Among its advantages are that it can be given as an out-patient treatment, and that most patients are able to tolerate it without undue side-effects. In order to succeed, the treatment has to be custom designed for each patient, to ensure that a high dose of x-rays can be given to the prostate gland, while as low a dose as possible is given to the surrounding tissues. The treatment planning to achieve this usually involves a CT scan, which gives a cross-sectional image of the prostate and surrounding tissues, and provides information that the radiotherapist can feed directly into the planning computer. This is why a planning CT scan may be needed, even if a patient has already had a previous CT or MRI scan performed. The radiotherapy physicist can then use a planning computer to work out the best x-ray beam size and arrangement. A frequently used technique employs three 'fields' (or beams) – one from the front, and two from each side. Typically, a patient, lying on his back on a treatment couch, is treated first with the machine

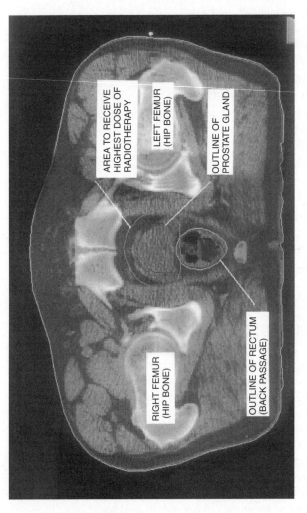

AREA TO RECEIVE
HIGHEST DOSE OF
RADIOTHERAPY

LEFT FEMUR
(HIP BONE)

OUTLINE OF
PROSTATE GLAND

RIGHT FEMUR
(HIP BONE)

OUTLINE OF RECTUM
(BACK PASSAGE)

Figure 4.1 The appearance of the prostate gland as viewed in the course of radiotherapy planning. Two outlines have been drawn using the planning computer. One encircles the prostate gland itself and the other, generated by the computer, adds a margin of 1 cm to this, in all directions except behind the prostate, where the margin is reduced to 5 mm to minimize the amount of the rectum in the radiotherapy field.

shining the x-ray beam at him from the front, and then swinging round to do so from each side. Each treatment takes a few minutes – indeed, it takes longer to ensure that a patient is in the correct position (to within millimetres) than it does to administer the treatment itself. This is repeated, on a daily basis (usually excluding weekends) for between 4 and 8 weeks (depending on the exact details of the technique, which vary between hospitals).

New radiotherapy technology – conformal therapy

Conventionally, radiotherapy planning makes use of two-dimensional images from a CT scan – in other words, pictures of the body in cross-section. From these pictures, a three-dimensional image of the prostate, tumour, and surrounding tissues can be built up. However, until very recently, a limitation of radiotherapy was that the head of a linear accelerator (the part from which the x-rays come into the open air) was rectangular in shape. Its jaws could move to give an x-ray beam of different sizes, but it would only be either square or rectangular. The area of the body which received the highest dose would thus be cylindrical in shape; however, tumours, prostates, and normal parts of the body are not cylindrical, but are irregular in shape.

Conformal radiotherapy uses an x-ray head which produces a beam which is not only irregular in shape, but which can be made into any shape that the therapist may desire. This makes use of a so-called multi-leaf collimator, which divides the jaws into a series of 'mini-jaws' that can be opened and shut independently of each other and to an independent extent. The result is that treatment can be better tailored to an individual's shape and size, plus the position and shape of the prostate/tumour. Although this has been used primarily as a way of reducing the side-effects of radiotherapy, it could also be a means whereby a higher dose of radiation can be given, at the cost of a similar rate of side-effects compared to conventional treatment, but with a higher chance of tumour control. This possibility is currently being investigated in a UK clinical trial.

This can reduce, but does not abolish side effects. Patients undergoing radiotherapy feel nothing at all while the machine is switched on. However, over the whole 4–8-week course of treatment, side-effects do occur, and these need to be discussed. The side-effects of radiotherapy can be divided into acute side-effects (those that occur during and immediately after the individual's radiotherapy) and late side-effects (those that occur months or even years after the radiotherapy has been completed).

Acute side-effects The urethra, which carries urine out of the bladder, passes right through the centre of the prostate gland. Inflammation of the urethra and bladder during a course of radiotherapy causes discomfort when passing urine, and the passing of urine more frequently. Because the prostate gland is so closely associated with the rectum (back passage), radiotherapy to the prostate gland inevitably involves giving a certain dose of radiation to the rectum. This results in a degree of inflammation, which manifests itself as diarrhoea, perhaps even with the passage of a small amount of blood. These side-effects usually start after about 2 weeks of radiotherapy, and can worsen over the remaining period. Generally, they settle around 4–6 weeks after the end of the course of treatment. In addition, during radiotherapy, patients may be more tired than usual. Diarrhoea can be managed with medication or with modification of diet, and urinary problems with fluids and sometimes antibiotics.

Long-term side-effects Uncommonly, the acute side-effects either fail to settle, or, cruelly, settle initially and then return after 6 months to 2 years. For such side-effects to be significant enough to interfere with a man's life is uncommon, doing so in 1–5 per cent of patients. However, for those patients in whom it occurs, it is worrying as such side-effects may be permanent. They respond to some degree to other treatments, but they may not go away completely. In addition, 40 per cent or more of men who are potent before radiotherapy may become impotent by 5 years after treatment. Incontinence following external beam radiotherapy is rare except in men who have had a previous TURP.

Brachytherapy in prostate cancer

Modern brachytherapy is a two-stage procedure. The first stage is to use transrectal ultrasound to measure the prostatic volume and to use data obtained to plan the number and positioning of radioactive sources, in an attempt to deliver a homogeneous dose of radiation to the prostate. The second stage involves the sources being inserted into the pre-planned position, through a needle under general anaesthetic. Usually, these needles are inserted through the perineal skin between the legs. Implants can be either removed or left in permanently, and in the UK most are permanent. Brachytherapy should theoretically have an advantage, in terms of damage to adjacent structures, such as the rectum and the nerves that were alongside the prostate. The disadvantage is that the area extending more than 3 or 4 mm outside the prostate capsule will not be irradiated, so any stray cancer cells present may not be treated. Not every patient is suitable for brachytherapy – for example, some centres will not use it to treat patients who have undergone a previous TURP.

Complications

Patients can develop significant urinary symptoms (see above) following prostate brachytherapy. In some series, between 4 and 8 per cent of patients required catheterization or cystoscopy in the weeks following brachytherapy. Bowel complications occur in less than 2 per cent of patients receiving implants as the sole treatment, and incontinence in up to 1 per cent.

Surgery

Surgical removal of a cancer is a well-established treatment for many types of cancer. In the case of prostate cancer, the operation removes the entire prostate, and not just the cancer. It must be stressed that a TURP does not do this – it merely removes the central 'core' of the prostate. Prostate cancers occur in other regions of the prostate, and there may be several separate tumours within the prostate gland. There are two main disadvantages of surgery: first, incontinence (being unable to control the flow of urine), and second, loss of sexual potency. In 1982, Patrick Walsh in the Johns Hopkins University in Baltimore, USA, developed a technique of removing the prostate but sparing the nerves which control erections. However, it must be emphasized that not every patient is suitable for this approach, though for suitable patients there is an operation where sexual ability is not necessarily lost.

Radical surgery is reserved for men whose disease it appears possible to remove completely, in the hope that this will cure the patient. It is also important that they will live long enough to benefit from any cure. This means that a patient must have a life expectancy of at least 10 years before considering radical surgery. The age and general health of the patient are also important. Age itself is not a bar to treatment, but the presence of other serious medical conditions can make surgery hazardous.

The operation

It is usual for surgery to be postponed for about 8 weeks after a needle biopsy of the prostate and for 12 weeks after a TURP (see later). In North America and in certain European countries, the patient may be given the opportunity to donate 2 or 3 units of blood, which can be transfused back into him if required. This is called autologous blood transfusion. Patients are usually advised to avoid taking aspirin and non-steroidal anti-inflammatory drugs, which interfere with the function of blood clotting. The anaesthetist will discuss the type of anaesthetic, which may be a general or spinal anaesthetic.

The incision is made from just above the pubic bone, to the umbilicus (tummy button). The prostate is then removed through the abdomen and the remaining bladder is joined on to the end of the urethra. The patient is normally allowed a clear liquid diet on the first postoperative day, building up to a regular diet on the third day. There may be suction drains coming from separate areas of the abdomen and these are removed when they stop discharging.

A catheter will have been placed in the bladder and the patient goes home with the catheter in position, returning 3 weeks after the procedure for removal.

Complications

The death rate is low and is of the order of 0.2 per cent. Complications at operation are bleeding, damage to the obturator nerve (supplying muscles in the leg), injury to the rectum and occasionally injury to the ureter.

Less than 10 per cent of men are significantly incontinent after surgery. However, the figure may be higher than this and figures of between 25 and 30 per cent are reported although most commonly this is minor and may improve. Patients over 65 appear to have a greater risk of incontinence. Continence should return in most men by 12 months, with over half achieving continence within 3 months. Should incontinence continue, treatments are available to deal with this.

Where the nerve bundles have been preserved, potency should return in at least 50 per cent of men. Viagra (sildenafil) or apomorphine (Uprima) are effective in some patients where potency has not been achieved (see Chapter 11).

The perineal operation

This operation, although less popular world wide, is achieving greater popularity. It is performed in the crutch, below the scrotum and does not require a large cut on the abdomen. Blood loss is much less and patients return home sooner. There is debate as to whether it preserves the nerves as well as the open operation. Continence rates appear to be similar to those of the open operation, as is the control of cancer.

5
Screening

Why is screening for prostate cancer so controversial? To many people, it seems obvious that, in order to cure more men of prostate cancer, screening should enable a diagnosis to be made at the earliest possible stage, and should be done as a matter of course. Despite this, the reluctance of the UK government to institute a screening programme seems implacable. To understand the scientific – as opposed to the political – reasons behind this, we must look at both the advantages and the disadvantages of prostate cancer screening.

Before doing this, we briefly consider what screening involves. The most common practice is to use a blood test for PSA (prostate-specific antigen, see Chapter 1). In patients whose PSA level is elevated, further tests are performed. This will involve a consultation with a specialist, usually a urologist. He will perform a rectal examination (see Chapter 1), and subsequently an ultrasound test, which is carried out using a probe inserted into the rectum. This may or may not identify an abnormality in the prostate. In either event, it will be necessary to biopsy the prostate gland, which is carried out with a needle that passes through the rectum and into the gland. If the ultrasound identifies an abnormality, it will be biopsied, but if no abnormality is seen, the prostate will need to be biopsied 'blindly'. Usually, six or eight biopsy samples are taken – from the upper, middle, and lower part of the gland on each side. It may be that, in the future, even more samples are taken. This can be an unpleasant procedure, and a proportion of men develop an infection following this (though treating all patients who have a biopsy with antibiotics reduces this). If the biopsy shows evidence of prostate cancer, the treatment options then need to be discussed. If the biopsy does not show prostate cancer, there are a number of options for the next step, which very much depend on the overall picture. It may be necessary to repeat the transrectal ultrasound and biopsy in the future. This would particularly be the case if the biopsy showed changes that in themselves were not cancerous, but which are known to precede cancer in some men (this is *prostatic intraepithelial neoplasia*, or *PIN*).

It may be clear by now that the blood test for PSA, the initial test in the screening process, is the simplest one to undertake (from both the patient's and from the doctor's point of view). The subsequent tests are more complicated, and more unpleasant. They are also not perfect, in the sense that they may not give a definitive answer to the question 'Have I got prostate cancer?' or may even give the wrong answer. This is part of the reason for the controversy.

Let us now consider the advantages and disadvantages of screening. The *advantages* are:

- that it may allow a cure of an otherwise fatal disease;
- that, by identifying a cancer at an early stage, treatment might be more straightforward than if it had been discovered later;
- that introducing a screening service would also introduce well-organized networks of specialists involved in treating prostate cancer.

These are pretty big advantages, especially the first, so why the controversy?

The first disadvantage of screening is that we do not know if it works. There is, therefore, the possibility that it does not work (or rather that, if a national screening programme were introduced, it would not reduce deaths from prostate cancer). This might matter less were it not for the cost of screening (estimated by one expert at £1.3 billion per year in the UK, which could not currently be met by the UK National Health Service, and which insurance companies in the USA struggle to support). Third, as has been discussed, in its present form it may not give the correct answer, or even a definitive answer. Quite apart from the stress, and the unpleasantness of the investigations when a definite answer is given, the extra psychological stress of screening in general (especially when it has to be repeated) is now known to be real, and is very well described. Finally, even when we know that a patient has prostate cancer, we may not know what the best form of treatment is, or even whether it needs treatment at all (see Chapter 4). Furthermore, treatments have complications (Chapter 4). It is beyond doubt that, if we screened all men, some would suffer serious complications from a treatment which they never needed in the first place (see also Chapter 3).

One approach to this dilemma is to perform a randomized trial of screening. This would involve randomly allocating men to screening or no screening (see Chapter 9), and comparing the death rates from prostate cancer in the two groups. Such studies are currently under way in the USA and in Europe. In the UK, a study termed the 'ProtecT study' is identifying healthy men who are invited to undergo a combination of PSA testing plus (if they turn out to have prostate cancer) a randomized study (see Chapter 9) of active monitoring versus radical prostatectomy versus radical radiotherapy (it must be stressed that this study is limited to nine UK centres and is not nationwide). It will, however, be many years before the results are known.

6
Hormone therapy

Prostate cancer requires the male sexual hormone, testosterone, in order to continue growing. It has been known for over 50 years that by interfering with or depriving the tumour of testosterone, its cells will die. Testosterone deprivation (also called 'androgen deprivation', or simply 'hormone therapy') will keep a tumour under control for some time – maybe for some years. However, it usually does not completely eradicate it, but rather, reaches a state of 'détente' between the body and the tumour. The most obvious means of androgen deprivation, is to remove the testicles.

Hormone therapy may be used at various stages of the disease. Some patients will have hormone therapy prior to, during, and even after a course of radical radiotherapy (see Chapter 4). Hormone therapy may be used by itself in patients with locally advanced disease (see Chapter 7), or metastatic disease.

The first effective drug treatment for prostate cancer was a compound called 'diethylstilboestrol' (DES) or 'stilboestrol'. This is an effective treatment for prostate cancer, but is less commonly used now because of its side-effects, particularly heart disease and strokes, and gynaecomastia (enlargement of the male breast). In recent years, there has been more interest in using stilboestrol at low doses, where the side-effects may be far less.

Hormone therapy cause side-effects similar to the menopause in women and this includes hot flushes (called hot flashes in North America), and sexual problems, such that nearly all men will become impotent and lose sexual interest. In addition, some forms of hormone therapy given by tablet can cause liver problems and enlargement of the male breasts (gynaecomastia).

Gonadorelin (gonadotrophin, or LH-RH) analogues

The pituitary gland, which lies at the base of the brain, controls the production of the male sexual hormone and other hormones. It does this by releasing messenger hormones called follicle-stimulating hormone (FSH) and luteinizing hormone (LH). Gonadorelin analogues interfere with the production of these hormones. They cause an initial stage of stimulation and then a reduction of their production. During the initial stage there may be an increase of production of testosterone by the testicles and in some patients this can lead to an increased growth of the tumour, which is called 'tumour flare'. This can, for example, increase bone pain and even lead to spinal problems.

In view of this, where there is a possibility that this may occur, another drug called a 'anti-androgen', such as cyproterone acetate or flutamide, may be given at least 3 days before the gonadorelin analogue is given. They would normally be continued for up to 3 weeks after the first injection.

Various preparations of gonadorelin

These all have their advantages and disadvantages. In the UK, the most commonly prescribed forms are goserelin and leuprorelin.

Buserelin

This is given by an injection under the skin in the abdomen every 8 hours and then by nasal spray, one spray into each nostril six times daily.

Suprefact

This is given by an injection under the skin in the abdomen every 8 hours and then by nasal spray, one spray into each nostril six times daily.

Goserelin (Zoladex)

This is given by injection every 28 days. There is also a preparation available (Zoladex LA), which is given every 12 weeks.

Leuprorelin acetate

This is available as a subcutaneous injection, given either every 4 weeks or every 3 months. A long-acting preparation may be given every 12 weeks.

Decapeptyl

This is by intramuscular injection every 4 weeks.

Anti-androgens

There are three main anti-androgens, which act in a way different from the gonadorelins. They interfere with the action of testosterone, rather than by reducing its levels. Because they act in this way, they can be given to cover the period of potential flare when gonadorelins are started.

Cyproterone acetate (Cyprostat; Androcur)

This drug, usually given as 300 mg in two to three divided doses daily, can damage the liver directly and liver function tests are required before treatment. It is not normally recommended for long-term treatment of prostate cancer, due to the reported side-effects.

Flutamide

This causes gynaecomastia (enlargement of the male breast) and can also cause diarrhoea and various other abdominal symptoms. It can also cause damage to the liver. It is occasionally used in patients where they wish to preserve sexual function. It is not clear whether it is quite as effective as the other agents in controlling cancer, but any differences are probably small. Patients often decide on this drug after discussion.

Bicalutamide (Casodex)

This is given as 150 mg once daily, by tablet. Side-effects include hot flushes and gynaecomastia. It may preserve sexual interest more than other drugs, but is not usually used by itself for patients with metastases, unless they are part of a drug trial.

Coping with side-effects

Patients should be reassured that hormonal treatment will not make them become effeminate. Although beard growth may be slowed up, and there may be some loss of body hair, none of these treatments will cause hair loss on the head. To those not 'in the know', a patient on hormone therapy will look completely normal. They should also be reassured that their voice will not change.

Hot flushes

Hot flushes can vary from being trivial, to quite disabling. It is rare that treatment has to be discontinued. These symptoms are very similar to those that happen to women when they are going through the change of life. Where flushes are troublesome, they can be easily treated with a small dose of cyproterone acetate, by tablet or using a drug called 'Provera' (medroxyprogesterone acetate).

7

Locally advanced disease and advanced disease

Locally advanced disease

This somewhat alarming term is used to describe a prostate cancer which, although it has spread to the tissues immediately outside the prostate gland itself, has not given rise to detectable disease elsewhere, such as in lymph glands or bones. It is a more serious situation than disease confined to the prostate gland, for a number of reasons:

- It suggests that the type of cancer is likely to be one that would, untreated, cause problems to the patient (see Chapter 3). Hence, it is more likely to need treatment, although this is not always the case (for example, a slowly progressing tumour in an elderly patient with other significant illnesses might never cause problems within that patient's lifetime).

- It suggests that, if treated, surgery (a radical prostatectomy) would be unlikely to remove all of the tumour, and other options (hormone therapy, radiotherapy – see below) are more likely to be appropriate.

- It is associated with a higher risk, at a later date, of developing prostate cancer in other parts of the body than is the case in patients with prostate cancer confined to the prostate gland.

None of the above suggests that the situation is hopeless – very far from it – although it is clearly more serious than in some other patients with prostate cancer. It does, however, define the range of treatment and management options that might be appropriate.

There are three main options for the management of locally advanced disease: watchful waiting, radiotherapy, and hormone therapy.

Hormone therapy for locally advanced and metastatic disease

Hormone therapy is the mainstay of treatment for locally advanced and advanced prostate cancer. It is described more fully in Chapter 6, but some aspects of it will be reviewed again here. All forms of hormone therapy are designed to interfere with the male hormone, testosterone, which characteristically 'feeds' prostate cancer cells. Hormone therapy is sometimes referred to by other terms, such as androgen ablation therapy, anti-androgen therapy, or androgen deprivation therapy; it all means the same thing.

There are three main ways of administering hormone therapy in locally advanced disease. They are all, broadly, as effective as each other, and the choice between them is made by a combination of the physician's preference and the patient's preference.

- The oldest form of treatment is the bilateral orchidectomy (removal of both testicles, leaving the capsule of the testicle and the other contents of the scrotum intact).

- An alternative to orchidectomy is a monthly injection (or, more recently, a 3-monthly, very long-acting injection), of a drug which causes the level of testosterone in the blood to fall. This drug is called a 'LH-RH' (luteinizing hormone-releasing hormone) 'agonist', or, alternatively, a 'gonadotrophin-releasing hormone' (GnRH) agonist or a gonadorelin. These drugs are analogues of the hormone, LH-RH, which is produced in the brain, and which stimulates the pituitary gland to produce the hormone LH. This, in turn, stimulates the testicles to produce testosterone. Because of the way in which these drugs act, they cause a transient but dramatic *rise* in testosterone levels for the first week or two after they are started, followed by a profound and dramatic fall in testosterone levels, equivalent to those seen after an orchidectomy.

- It is also possible to interfere with the actions of testosterone with tablets, called oral anti-androgens, which, although they do not reduce the level of testosterone in the blood, block its actions on cells (normal and cancerous). It has been claimed that oral anti-androgens may have fewer side-effects than other forms of hormone therapy, but not all specialists agree on this, and some feel that more data are needed to support this assertion.

Irrespective of the mode of hormone therapy, the important 'bottom line' is that the response rates (i.e. the percentage of patients whose tumours will shrink significantly, and/or whose blood PSA levels will fall significantly) are in excess of 85 per cent. Many of these responses are so-called complete responses, i.e. the tumour in and around the prostate gland shrinks to undetectable levels, and the PSA level falls to within the normal range. They can also be long-lasting in some patients who continue hormone therapy long-term, keeping the disease under control for some years. As with hormone therapy for metastatic (advanced) disease, such responses cannot, unfortunately, be guaranteed to last for the patient's lifetime. Most importantly, to the patient with symptoms from an enlarged prostate (such as frequency of urination, discomfort when urinating), hormone therapy will often result in a dramatic resolution or improvement in those symptoms (as discussed earlier, see Chapter 6).

However, as with hormone therapy administered for other stages of the illness, patients may suffer from the same side-effects, as discussed in more detail in

Chapter 6. These include impotence, a loss of libido (sexual desires), hot flushes, some tendency to put on weight, and some reduction in the amount of facial and body hair. Contrary to what is learned from one's schoolfellows, hormone therapy does not cause the voice to become higher, or to grow breasts, although some degree of breast enlargement may occur with some oral anti-androgens (see Chapter 6 for a fuller discussion of this). It is partly because of the side-effects that, in some patients, hormone therapy may be administered for a limited time – either a few months, or a few years, rather than indefinitely. However, more commonly, in patients with locally advanced disease who are treated with hormone therapy, it is continued indefinitely, though it has to be said that we do not know for certain whether it is necessary to do so.

Radiotherapy

Radiotherapy (radiation therapy, or x-ray therapy), as discussed in more detail in Chapter 4, consists of the use of high energy x-rays (which are a form of radiation), which cause damage to, and kill, cancer cells. They also damage and kill normal cells, but normal cells have a greater ability to repair radiation damage. Consequently, it is possible, by carefully administering radiotherapy, to completely destroy a cancerous tumour without also destroying the normal tissues which surround it.

Radiotherapy is sometimes used, in patients with locally advanced disease, to treat the prostate gland plus the surrounding tissues, thus encompassing all the tumour in a way that would not be possible with surgery. The technical aspects of radiotherapy, plus a discussion of its side-effects, are covered in Chapter 5.

Combined hormone therapy plus radiotherapy

There is a growing tendency among specialists to add hormone therapy to the treatment of patients who are receiving radiotherapy, based on studies that have suggested that the addition of hormone therapy improves the results of radiotherapy. The duration of hormone therapy used in this context varies considerably, from a few months to several years, and there is no consensus as to what is optimum.

What is unknown is whether, for patients being treated with long-term hormone therapy, the addition of radiotherapy is beneficial. There is a subtle, but important difference between this question, and the question posed above:

• *In patients for whom the specialist feels that radiotherapy is definitely required,* there is evidence that additional hormone therapy (short- or long-term) might be beneficial.

• *In patients for whom the specialist feels that long-term hormone therapy is definitely required,* who may differ from the above group in a number of ways, there is no evidence that additional radiotherapy is beneficial. However, this possibility is currently being investigated in an international collaborative study, in which the UK is participating.

Active monitoring/watchful waiting

Not every patient with locally advanced disease needs treatment, for the reasons already given. The decision to treat or not to treat is one of the hardest that a doctor and a patient have to make. Certain factors may sway either party in one direction rather than another, but this includes a patient's own preference. There is no 'right' or 'wrong' answer to this. No-one can say that a patient who opts not to have his locally advanced prostate cancer treated is making a wrong decision, although, if there is evidence that it is a potentially active tumour, he may well need treatment for symptoms sooner or later.

TURP in locally advanced cancer of the prostate

In the same way that a benign prostate enlarges and causes blockage of the urethra, a malignant prostate can enlarge and cause the same type of symptoms. Curiously, this can happen even when the disease appears to be under control. Where this occurs, the surgeon may suggest a TURP. This may not be the first time that a patient has had the operation and when cutting through further tissue, relief can easily be obtained. Sometimes the operation needs to be performed a number of times and usually produces significant relief.

Where a patient is not fit enough for a further TURP, then a tube or catheter may be suggested on a long-term basis. This has the effect of allowing the bladder to drain and avoids an operation.

Treatments for advanced or metastatic cancer

Orchidectomy

This means the removal of the testicles. The testicles produce 90 per cent of the male sex hormones and the advantage of this operation means that hormone treatment is started at an early stage and also avoids injections or remembering to take drug treatments.

It is, of course, not reversible. It formerly enjoyed great popularity because it is a relatively cheap option, avoiding expensive drug bills over a period of time.

The disadvantages are obvious, in that a surgical operation and anaesthetic are required.

It appears to work as well as any of the drugs and it is really a matter of personal preference as to which is undertaken. It will completely abolish sexual function.

The incision is made, usually through the scrotum, which is the bag that contains the testicles. Sometimes the surgeon will carry out a subcapsular orchidectomy, which leaves a small amount of tissue in the scrotum.

Hormone therapy

This has been discussed in detail above, and in Chapter 6. Exactly the same considerations apply to patients with metastatic disease, except that hormone therapy is usually given for an indefinite period of time.

Treatments for patients whose disease worsens after hormone therapy

This is a serious situation, but one in which an increasing number of treatments are becoming available. This may be termed 'hormone failed', or 'hormone refractory' disease.

Despite these names, a *second-line hormone treatment* is often used, and may produce further responses. There is no 'best buy' in this situation, and the choice of drugs may be made from any of the options discussed in Chapter 6. However, following an orchidectomy or gonadorelin therapy, the usual second-line hormone is an oral anti-androgen or stilboestrol. Steroid therapy, using drugs such as prednisolone or dexamethasone, may work just like other forms of hormone therapy. Disappointingly, second-line responses are often neither as good, nor as long as first-line responses.

Patients with metastatic disease commonly have secondaries in the bones, which can be painful. *External beam radiotherapy*, given as a short course (e.g. five sessions) or even as a single treatment, is effective at relieving bone pain, with minimal side-effects. This is a different situation from the longer course of radiotherapy described in Chapter 4. An alternative is to use a radioactive drug such as strontium, or samarium, given by a single injection as an out-patient. This is as good as external beam radiotherapy in relieving pain, and in some patients may have the added advantage of preventing further pain in the short to medium term. Patients can return home after a strontium injection, though some minor precautions will need to be taken for a couple of weeks. In addition, a wide range of pain-killing drugs are now available, and can be given with the hope of major or complete pain relief in every patient. There is no reason for a patient with metastatic disease to suffer pain without having it adequately treated. Morphine is a superb pain killer, given for this reason and because of its flexibility in terms of dose, and *not because using morphine means a patient is 'terminal'*. Addiction does not occur when morphine is given for cancer pain.

Recently, there has been an upsurge of interest in the use of *chemotherapy* in some patients with metastatic prostate cancer. This would usually be given as a series of injections as an out-patient. In the old days, chemotherapy had a fearsome reputation for its side-effects, but especially for causing vomiting. These days, vomiting is controlled or abolished with the use of new, powerful anti-sickness drugs. Some degree of hair loss can occur, and, depending on the exact drugs used, patients may be more susceptible to infection, bleeding, or bruising. This would need to be discussed in detail with the specialist before embarking on chemotherapy, but trials now suggest that some patients do benefit from this approach with no detriment – and even an improvement – in their quality of life.

Many other drugs are appearing on the scene. *Bisphosphonates* are a class of drug that may reduce the bone destruction that cancer secondaries can cause. There is some evidence that they might prove to be of value in prostate cancer. A range of newer drugs is being tested in clinical trials, and the repertoire is only going to increase in the future.

8
Alternative treatments

The Medical Establishment can frequently appear as very authoritarian. When patients suggest alternative treatments, they are often greeted with a shrug, but rarely with any genuine interest on behalf of the physician. There are a number of physicians who are prepared to entertain alternative treatments, but almost all reputable physicians will suggest alternative treatments as an addition to standard treatment, and not as a substitute.

It must be remembered that treatments that are orthodox today may have been considered alternative in the past. New treatments need to be scrutinized very carefully, to assess whether they work and whether they are safe. Many alternative treatments are not regulated and are often not obtainable in many countries.

It is natural that patients should grasp at straws and many of the practitioners in alternative medicine would appear to be very articulate and caring. Almost all genuinely believe in the efficacy of their treatments and occasionally they may appear as renegades, claiming that standard medicine and doctors do not take them seriously.

A sensible position will allow patients to pursue any alternative treatment that they may wish, as long is it is not harmful. It should be remembered that some of the alternative treatments are both unproven and occasionally dangerous. Many of the alternative therapies would not be acceptable because they have not been proven to work and have not been subjected to the rigorous analysis of randomized controlled trials. Conventional medicine does not know everything, however, and as long as the treatment is not harmful, then why shouldn't a patient try it, if he wishes? It is important to discuss this with the doctor first, however; the individual should beware the alternative practioner who tries to persuade him not to do so.

Seeking some of these treatments arises out of a sense of guilt. Patients may feel that some defect in their behaviour, emotion, or religious faith may have brought a visitation of disease. Sir Ludwig Guttman asserted that happy people do not get cancer. He was laughed at initially, but it is now perceived that the nervous system has a much more profound effect on the body than was originally realized.

There has been considerable interest recently of a visualization technique, to increase the effectiveness of the immune system. These techniques initially exploit the idea that a healthy mind will produce a healthy body. Counselling, hypnosis, and biofeedback can be used to promote greater emotional and spiritual well-being. It is occasionally claimed that these techniques change the course of an illness and induce remission.

There is no doubt that challenging life events, such as bereavement, lower the lymphocyte count and so there may be a respectable scientific basis for pursuit of these types of treatment.

Non-drug drugs

In the course of development of new drugs, many plant extracts, fungi, etc., are analysed. Practitioners will claim that the use of one of their new agents will make a great difference to the cancer or to the patient's well-being.

Perhaps some of these new agents may prove to be of benefit, but one may care to ask why conventional drug companies have not bought them up, since they would make a fortune if they found a cure for prostate cancer.

In an experimental sense, there are a variety of newer agents being tried and, for example, shark cartilage, which is a natural food substance, is being studied carefully. It remains to be seen, however, whether it will produce any real benefit for patients.

Immune therapies

There have been a variety of immune therapies produced. Some of these are potentially toxic, however, and care must be taken with any physician who is not prepared to test his theories using standard controlled trials.

Herbal therapies

Various herbs have been used as potential treatments, but once again, comments about new agents above hold true. One that deserves special mention is PC-SPES, previously available in the USA. This has been investigated in clinical trials, and it appears that it has hormone-like effects, and, indeed, probably works just like conventional hormone therapy. Whether it is actually 'better' than current conventional hormone therapy could only be tested in a randomized trial (see Chapter 9).

Metabolic therapies

This essentially applies a detoxification of the body and anti-cancer diets, based on what are perceived as more natural foods, e.g. vitamins, minerals, and enzymes, which are alleged to cleanse the body. They are also alleged to repair damaged tissue and stimulate immune function. The body is, of course, quite capable of doing this on its own and there is no evidence that immune function and prostate cancer are diminished.

Immune function certainly reduces as patients get older, but it has been disappointing that immune approaches to tumour therapy have not yielded much practical value.

Once again, the patient who wishes to try these diets should feel free to do so, if they are safe, and who knows?

As far as diet is concerned, there is no real evidence that modifying diet after developing cancer makes any difference. Our own advice would be for the individual to take the advice of a physician in whom he has confidence.

9
Clinical trials

What is a 'clinical trial'? Its very name conjures up images – perhaps a courtroom? Trials and Tribulations? Using patients as 'guinea pigs'? However, in the development of cancer treatments, clinical trials have played a vital role. Without them, we would lack many of the important cancer treatments that are now available. It is well known that the use of clinical trials to test and develop new cancer treatments is widely supported by the majority of the population, and yet relatively few people are prepared to enter a clinical trial themselves – perhaps rightly? Whatever the reasons, or the rights and wrongs, it is a fact that, in the UK, only some 5 per cent of cancer patients are ever treated within the context of a clinical trial, and for prostate cancer patients the figure is considerably lower than this. Before discussing the advantages and disadvantages of clinical trials, we first need to discuss what a clinical trial is, and how it is designed.

Design and conduct of clinical trials of cancer treatment

Conventionally, cancer treatments are evaluated in trials which are classified as phase I, II, or III studies. Phase I and II studies apply particularly to new drugs that are being introduced, and phase III studies apply to a range of treatment options including radiotherapy, drug therapy, and hormone therapy. Phase III studies involve the comparison of two or more treatment strategies. In prostate cancer, there have been relatively few phase I and II studies compared with other cancer types, but this situation is gradually changing as new treatments are being developed.

Phase I studies

In a phase I study, a new drug is tested in patients with a range of cancers, whose illness is active, and who have already received all conventional anti-cancer treatments. More rarely, such a study may be done in healthy volunteers. Its aim is to discover the correct dose of the new drug, and to obtain an understanding of its side-effects and characteristics when used in humans. Usually this means starting the drug at a very low dose – defined by laboratory studies – and gradually increasing the dose until side-effects prevent any further increase (the so called 'dose-limiting toxicity' has been defined). Although it is hoped that a new drug in a phase I study will demonstrate anti-cancer activity – and such activity is always closely looked for and monitored – it is not in itself the primary goal, which is to define the correct dose and means of administration of the drug. More detailed study of anti-cancer activity is the remit of the phase II study.

Phase II studies

Phase II studies depend on the outcome of a phase I study, in that the starting point is that the best dose schedule is already worked out. Patients with a particular type of cancer – for example, prostate cancer – whose illness is active and who have already received all available conventional anti-cancer treatments, are then treated with the new agent, and they are closely monitored for signs of anti-cancer activity. It is particularly at this stage of investigation that the promise of new agents might first become evident. If such promise is demonstrated, the drug will proceed to phase III studies. If not, as unfortunately is the case in the majority of new agents, it is unlikely to be developed further in that particular cancer type.

Phase III studies – the randomized controlled trial (RCT)

Phase III studies involve a formal comparison of two or more treatment strategies, using single drugs, combinations of drugs, or combinations of treatment types (e.g. radiotherapy, hormone therapy). An important feature of these studies is that the selection of treatment is neither up to the patient, nor the doctor, but is decided at random by an outside source (e.g. a computer in a trials office). This is why such studies are referred to as 'randomized trials', and it is this aspect of them which is most perplexing to patients – and to doctors.

Why 'randomize'?

The reason for randomization is to eliminate bias. Everybody is biased – doctors, patients, nurses – to a greater or a lesser extent. It might be argued, however, that, as long as the patients are well matched, they should be allowed to choose a treatment option freely in a trial – as should their doctors. Let us examine the reasons why this is not the case.

Imagine a new treatment – called wondermycin – which is to be given alongside hormone therapy for prostate cancer. This treatment has been designed by Dr Bonehead, who is conducting a trial comparing the survival rates of patients treated with hormone therapy alone, or hormone therapy plus wondermycin, and he decides not to use randomization.

The first patient, Mr Slim, comes to the out-patient clinic. He is aged 50, a keen athlete, does not smoke, and has had a very small prostate cancer diagnosed. Under the microscope his cancer did not look aggressive, and his PSA level is only slightly raised. Dr Bonehead decides that he is an ideal candidate for wondermycin therapy.

The second patient, Mr Hobb, sees Dr Bonehead. Unlike Mr Slim, he is 78, is a heavy smoker, and weighs 18 stone. He had a large, aggressive looking cancer diagnosed, and has a very high PSA level. Dr Bonehead decides that he should not be treated with wondermycin, but should receive hormone therapy alone.

Five years later, Dr Bonehead observes that Mr Slim is alive and well, but sadly, Mr Hobb died only 2 months after his visit to out-patients. He concludes that wonder-mycin is an effective treatment for prostate cancer, but is he right? Might Mr Hobb's demise not be related to his general fitness, or to his more aggressive disease, rather than being related to the fact that he did not receive wondermycin. Mr Slim and Mr Hobb were not compar-able – there was a bias on the part of Dr Bonehead in selecting the fittest patient for his new therapy.

Patients can also be biased. Had they been given the choice of treatment, Mr Slim might have opted for won-dermycin, as an extra 'insurance' against his cancer returning, whereas Mr Hobb might have decided against it because he already had many hospital appointments, was already taking 10 types of tablets every day, and did not want to take any more, or to have any extra hospital visits.

These are biases, which, it could be argued, we can broadly identify, and perhaps do something about. The problem is that for every source of bias that is obvious, there tend to be others that are not obvious, and that may only become apparent many years later. These factors may be biological, e.g. characteristics of an illness associated with a particular activity or background, that we don't know about. They may be similar to those discussed, but less obvious. For all these reasons, it is recognized that randomization is the best defence against sources of bias – known or unknown – interfering with the correct inter-pretation of a phase III study, and the randomized trial is regarded as the international gold standard by which a new treatment strategy is judged.

The benefits of clinical trials

Immediate benefits (to the trial participants)

As a broad generalization, patients benefit from being treated within the context of clinical trials, almost irrespective of what the particular trial is about. This has been shown in a number of studies, which have looked at the quality of care, and the survival of patients while treated within the context of a randomized trial. Not only is the quality of care generally better for patients while treated as part of clinical trial, but they tend to survive for a longer period of time than do comparable patients not treated in the context of a trial. There are probably many reasons for this, among them being that hospitals that participate in clinical trials do, by and large, have a very high standard of clinical practice. In addition, patients in a clinical trial are generally monitored more closely, and a have a closer relationship with clinical staff, than patients who are being treated 'routinely', outside of a trial setting.

It is impossible to guarantee that every patient will benefit in this manner, but the very least that can be said is that, by its very nature, the treatment package that a patient would receive within a clinical trial, would be the 'best' available, since no clinical trial would be permitted by the professional, research, or lay ethical bodies were this not to be the case.

Longer-term benefits (to mankind)

It goes without saying that no clinical trial would be permitted were it not attempting to answer some question that was of genuine and substantial importance. Previous questions which have been answered by randomized clinical trials include the treatment of breast cancer by a 'lumpectomy' rather than by a full mastectomy, the use of tamoxifen, and of chemotherapy to prolong the survival of women with breast cancer following their surgery, the use of newer forms of radiotherapy for the treatment of lung cancer (or, as we have seen, for high-dose conformal radiotherapy for prostate cancer), or in the the use of chemotherapy for other types of cancer including cancer of the colon. Many of these are now regarded as 'standard', yet none of them would currently be possible, had previous generations of patients not consented to take part in the randomized trials that tested them. There is always a certain element of altruism in taking part in clinical research. Indeed, many consent forms contain the phrase 'I understand that this trial may not be of benefit to me, but may be of benefit to other patients in the future'.

In the case of prostate cancer, there are more unanswered questions than there are in many other types of cancer. In almost no other area of common cancer is there such a great need for research, using clinical trials, to test and compare treatments in order to answer some of these questions. Despite this, it has proved to be harder to conduct clinical trials in prostate cancer than in many other types of cancer. This is changing, albeit slowly. Nonetheless, there are some very good reasons why it is difficult to conduct randomized trials in prostate cancer. Some of the treatments that need to be tested are very different in their nature, and in their implications to the patient. For example, the comparison of surgery, radiotherapy, and surveillance, is universally regarded as being one of the most important of the unanswered questions about the treatment of 'early' prostate cancer. For some patients, these treatment options are so different that it is difficult or impossible to accept the idea of being allocated one of them by a random process.

The next few years will tell us whether it is possible to conduct randomized trials into many of the aspects of prostate cancer treatment. If not, time may be running out, and both doctors and patients might have to accept that there are certain ideas that society has determined are best left unanswered. The philosophical implications of such a conclusion are of an enormity that goes far beyond the remit of this book.

The drawbacks of clinical trials

The hazards to participants

Just as no cancer treatment can be considered to be entirely without risk, no clinical trial can be considered to be entirely without risk. Many of the risks will consist of the standard side-effects and complications of cancer treatments, although if a new treatment is also be considered, it may have unrecognized problems that would only appear during the course of a clinical card. The essential point is that patients are made fully aware of the hazards of any clinical trial before they agree to participate. This is demanded by professional and research bodies, generally agreed by defining ethical and moral principles that were enshrined in the Helsinki Declaration.

If the risks cannot be entirely eliminated, then it is axiomatic that they must be acceptable. As a guiding principle, a doctor should not enter a patient into a clinical trial he would not himself be prepared to enter, or have a member of his family entered into. Clinical trials can only be undertaken if the doctor and the patient are comfortable with the design and the immediate implications of the actual trial.

The restrictions to doctors

In order to protect both doctors and patients, there are a number of restrictions placed of the launching and conduct of a clinical trial. Before trials can be considered, the scientific background has to be accepted by a respected scientific body, such as the UK Medical Research Council, Cancer Research UK, or the scientific committee of another medical charity. In addition, many hospitals have their own scientific committee which will scrutinize proposed new clinical trials to be undertaken, and this will include some of the very important studies of new drugs which have been designed by the pharmaceutical industry.

The process of scientific approval can be very long, and may involve the examination of the proposed trial by a succession of different committees in that organization. This applies particularly to the major cancer charities and the Medical Research Council. In some instances, this can take several years.

Having made the scientific case for undertaking a clinical trial, and having persuaded the professional bodies that it is morally and ethically right to do so, a trial has to be passed by a local, or a national ethical committee, made up of both care professionals and lay members. This body will also expect to be kept informed about progress of the trial, and, in due course, of trial results. Some research bodies, for example the Medical Research Council, also have their own internal data monitoring and ethical committee, which reviews the conduct of the trial, and provides an independent assessment as to whether the progress of the trial justifies its continuation. For example, if in a comparison of treatments, one treatment appears to be showing superior results to another, the data monitoring committee may order the cessation of trial on ethical grounds.

It's OK to say 'no'!

Having described the importance of clinical trials, and having recognized the safeguards which are built into them to protect both patients and doctors, it is worth repeating the statement that a clinical trial can only be undertaken if the doctor and the patient feel comfortable with it. This will not always be the case – every patient is different, and every individual will have his/her own bank of experience, concepts, and beliefs. Some patients will not wish to take part in clinical trials offered, and it is entirely proper that they should feel free not to do so. It is almost more important than all the safeguards, that patients who decline the offer of entering a clinical trial, should feel that the care that they will receive will be the best available, and that they can refuse (or even change their mind at a later date, having already entered a trial) without any worry as to the implications that this may have. A hospital taking part in a clinical trial is likely to have a very high standard of practice, and no doctor will take it as a personal insult if the patient does not want to take part in clinical research. Consent to take part in a clinical trial must be freely given, and an informed choice.

The media: publicity and 'hype'

Cancer research is 'big business'. Charities depend on the steady flow of income to maintain their research base, and cancer stories are always popular items for the media. On the basis that, in order to sell newspapers, there has to be a good story, it is unfortunately the case that a clinical study that suggests that a new treatment may be beneficial is more likely to find its way into the media than a study that suggests no particular benefit. Equally, there is a tendency on the part of the media to 'hype' a new cancer treatment, even if the research suggesting its possibilities is at a very early stage. The road to a new cancer treatment is a long and arduous one, and many treatments that look promising in the early stages of research turn out to be without benefit, or to offer no particular advantages over and above those of existing treatments.

Some cancer stories are genuinely 'big' stories. However, for the majority, there is a danger that the story will raise false hopes, and patients who are distressed, and therefore very vulnerable, will often want to explore anything new that is reported the media. The doctor's responsibility is to provide that patient with an honest appraisal of the scientific evidence relating to a particular story, and if a particular new treatment is either inappropriate or unavailable, then he must be told this honestly and sympathetically.

Parting shot – 'more' is not always 'better'!

One common clinical trial design is one in which the new treatment is added to an existing one, and this sort of design confers particular difficulties for patients. For example, an ongoing clinical trial in prostate cancer is investigating whether, for certain patients who are being treated with hormone therapy, the addition of radiotherapy is beneficial.

Why do this as a randomized clinical trial? Surely, it might be reasonably argued, if there is any suspicion that 'more' treatment might be better, it would be reasonable to simply add that treatment in. After all, the results of many treatments for cancer are unsatisfactory, and anything that might make them better is fully justified. Indeed, some people say that it is irresponsible not to simply add in whichever extra treatments are available, and that a failure to do so is merely another example of economic stringency.

This seemingly sensible argument rests on one assumption – that is, that additional treatment is only likely to be beneficial, and will not be harmful. Unfortunately, we already know that this is not the case. The best example of this has come from a detailed analysis of all studies examining the addition of radiotherapy to surgery for patients with lung cancer. This might be expected to be a situation where extra treatment could only benefit patients, but, rather surprisingly, the reverse was the case. The survival of patients who were treated with a combination of surgery plus radiotherapy was actually worse than the survival of patients treated with surgery alone. Modern cancer treatments are powerful, and we cannot simply add in the treatments without testing such a combination in a formal way.

10
Prostate cancer and sex

Sex is part of healthy living for all of us. The sexual urge decreases in most men with time. Nonetheless, it is well known that men can father children well into their 80s. A woman's interest in sex may decrease after the menopause, but this is not necessarily so. Most men who have prostate cancer are not in the first flush of youth and for some couples sexual activity may have virtually stopped in any case. For some men, even elderly men, the inability to have intercourse can be devastating. For others, it may not matter. Neither instance is 'right' or 'wrong'.

Impotence

Impotence can be both mental or physical. Impotence is defined as the inability to achieve and maintain a firm enough erection to permit penetration in intercourse.

Impotence can occur at any age group. It is probably true to say that most men have a period of impotence at some stage in their life. This can be caused by depression, bereavement, etc. As men get older, frequency of intercourse and penile rigidity gradually reduce. In some men, the male sexual hormone may decrease significantly with age.

Being given the diagnosis of cancer is, of course, unlikely to improve your sex life and it can take a number of months for patients to adjust to this knowledge. One reaction is that the patient thinks cancer has been visited upon him for some reason, perhaps due to previous sexual encounters or perceived bad conduct at some stage. A perception of being 'unclean' may develop and it is important that the spouse understands what may appear to be rejection. Another anxiety that male patients have is that they may pass on their disease in some way to their wives. This is just not possible and is not a reason to abstain from intercourse. Patients should also be reassured that sexual intercourse will not accelerate or alter the disease. Many of the treatments of prostate cancer will produce either complete or partial impotence and the consultant should have discussed this with each patient.

Although these questions can be embarrassing, one should not feel embarrassed asking the urologist. The urologist deals with many men for a wide variety of sexual problems and he may merely assume that an individual who does not enquire is not interested in asking.

Treatments

Viagra (sildenafil)

Of the various treatments available for impotence, one of the best known is Viagra (sildenafil). This probably does not work quite so well in patients with prostate cancer, but is certainly worth trying. The usual starting dose is 50 mg, as a tablet, taken about 1 hour before sexual activity. This may be reduced to 25 mg in elderly men and the largest single dose is 100 mg, which is available as a separate tablet. Erections may not occur spontaneously and genital manipulation may be required. It is recommended that the drug is not repeated for 24 hours. Sildenafil is contraindicated in men on glyceryl trinitrate (GTN) tablets or in patients with a recent history of stroke or heart attack. It should also be avoided in patients with low blood pressure and, rarely, in patients with disorders of the retina of the eye. This drug is not available on the NHS for all patients with erectile dysfunction, but is available for patients who have had treatment for prostate cancer, particularly those who have had radical prostatectomy or other forms of pelvic surgery. The side-effects include headache, flushing of the face, dizziness, and, in some people, disturbance of blue/green colour perception. Nasal congestion can also occur. It is important that if an erection lasts for more than 4 hours, urgent medical attention is sought.

Apomorphine

Apomorphine (Uprima) is a newer drug that has become available and is taken in a dose of 2 mg under the tongue. A 3 mg tablet is also available should the first dose not work.

Injections into the penis

Alprostadil is prostaglandin E_1. It is given by self-administered injection. Some preparations come as a powder, which has to be made up with fluid, which is also supplied. The injection is into the shaft of the penis. The initial dose is 5 μg, which may be increased up to 20 μg, with a maximum of 40 μg. It is recommended that this injection is used only once in one day and not more than two to three times in any one week. Special training must be given to patients before they use it.

Alprostadil (MUSE)

The dosage of the pellet, which is placed in the urethra at the opening of the penis, is 250 μg and it is recommended that this be used not more than twice in a 24-hour period.

Surgical implants

Very occasionally, patients may wish to explore the use of a penile implant. This can be either rigid or inflatable. It is our opinion that these devices may have a place, but it should be remembered that the enjoyment which is given is almost exclusively to the female and the insertion of these devices stops any attempt at further drug treatment.

There are a number of non-surgical devices, such as vacuum pumps, and this can be explored on request.

Questions and answers

Q. *What are the early symptoms of prostate cancer?*

A. Early prostate cancer does not usually have symptoms. Enlargement of the prostate can cause difficulty passing water, blood in the water and a reduction in urinary stream. This is usually caused by what is called benign enlargement of the prostate.

Q. *What is the difference between a tumour and cancer?*

A. A tumour involves enlargement of any group of cells within the body. Tumours can be benign or malignant. Benign tumours may cause problems locally by enlargement, such as reduction of urinary stream. They are not, however, malignant. Cancers have two properties, which cause them to be malignant. They can invade locally and they can spread to distant sites.

Q. *How do tumours kill people?*

A. Tumours can kill people by various mechanisms. First, they can run away with all the essential foodstuffs that the body requires and while the body is starving, the tumour is growing at the expense of its host. Second, tumours cause problems by growing in places where they cause local damage and obstruction, e.g. tumours growing within the central nervous system can cause problems with the circuitry of the nervous system. Secondary tumours growing in the liver can press on the bile ducts and cause jaundice. Third, tumours can produce substances, which cause the rest of the body to malfunction.

Q. *Can benign tumours become malignant?*

A. There is very little, if any, evidence to suggest that benign enlargement of the prostate turns into malignancy. Benign enlargement of the prostate is extremely common and most men will have some degree of this within their lives.

Q. *Why is cancer so common?*

A. The question really should be why with all the numbers of dividing cells within the body is cancer not more common? It tends to get more common as we get older and this is mainly due to DNA damage and also reaction to agents, such as viruses that subvert the normal pattern of cell replacement.

Q. *How quickly does the cancer grow?*

A. Different cancers grow at different rates. Some men's prostate may harbour it for many, many years, before it becomes clinically evident. Some unfortunate men have very aggressive forms of cancer and these can grow at a great rate and cause death within a very short space of time.

Q. *Can I catch cancer from someone?*

A. Prostate cancer is not transmitted either from male to female or male to male.

Q. *Does the body have natural defences against cancer?*

A. The body has a whole variety of defences against abnormal cell growth. The DNA, which is the construction plan for each cell, is kept within the nucleus of each cell. There are highly adapted packaging proteins for

DNA called histones, which package the DNA in clumps. The DNA itself has two chains, both of which are complementary, so it means that if one strand gets damaged, the opposite strand can still provide a template for the DNA to be replaced without change.

There are various enzymes, which control the defence of the DNA. If a cell becomes damaged, there is an actual mechanism to cause it to die and this is called apoptosis. If a cell becomes too much of a renegade, it can develop different cell coatings. The immune system constantly patrols the cells of the body and in many circumstances might pick up abnormal cells and kill them. It does this to control both cancer and also any bacteria, which enter the system.

Q. *Can I reduce the risk of prostate cancer?*

A. There is no foolproof way of reducing the risk. Although there is a slight association with smoking, it could not be said that smoking is strongly associated with prostate cancer. There are sufficient reasons, however, to give up smoking without looking at prostate cancer risk. A normal healthy diet should contain enough vitamins and antioxidants to prevent cancer.

If you are eating a normal healthy balanced diet, with enough fruit and vegetables, e.g. five items of fruit and vegetables per day, it should not be necessary to top up the level of vitamins occurring naturally. Small amounts of proprietary vitamins will not do any harm, but there are instances where particular vitamins, such as vitamin A, can in fact be harmful. Too much vitamin C predisposes you to develop stones in your urinary tract.

Q. *Is there a connection between cancer and emotional states?*

A. Sir Ludwig Guttman used to state that happy people do not get cancer. It was originally felt that he was making an unsupportable statement, despite his evidence in dealing with spinal injuries, and his comments were laughed at.

Nowadays we are not so sure. There is unquestionably a link between the immune system and positive attitudes. It can certainly be said that none of the emotional treatments do any harm and many people find it at worst a comfort in their time of trial.

In certain illnesses, visualization of the tumour has been thought to be helpful and there is a whole new science of psychobiology, where patients are given support to deal with their illness.

Q. *My father died of prostate cancer at age 55. Do I have an increased chance of developing the disease?*

A. Current evidence suggests a modest degree of increased risk with one close relative affected, increasing if more than one are affected. It is worthwhile discussing this further with the specialist, although it is unknown whether monitoring (or 'screening') are effective.

Q. *If there is an increased chance, should I be on a screening programme?*

A. The British Government has now decided that any patient wishing to have his PSA tested can have this done. It is important that this test is understood fully (*see* Chapters 2 & 3).

It is worth reflecting that patients are very keen to have a negative test, but in the small chance that they have a positive test, would they really wish to know, given that the treatment options are not clearly defined?

Q. *What are the options if screening indicates a rising PSA level?*

A. The options are:
  1. to do nothing and disregard it
  2. to have the PSA monitored
  3. to ask for a urological/oncological opinion

4. through a urologist or oncologist, ask for a transrectal ultrasound and biopsy, if it is felt appropriate.

Q. *What are the chances that there is spread of this disease?*

A. It rather depends on how advanced the disease is when it has been discovered. In the past almost 50 per cent of people had advanced disease, but now patients who are having their PSA tested are being identified at a much earlier stage.

Q. *Can the specialist tell if my cancer will spread?*

A. Unfortunately, it is not possible to tell with any certainty. Gleason scores that are higher indicate more likelihood of spread than those that are lower, but there is no one feature that tells us which is going to be a 'tiger' and which is going to be a 'pussycat'.

Q. *What is my life expectancy?*

A. This rather depends on how advanced your tumour is. It is comforting to note that many patients who were followed up in Scandinavia, who had in fact received no treatment, survived in excess of 10 years. They were perhaps lucky, but nonetheless, a diagnosis of prostate cancer does not indicate necessarily that it will be the cause of death.

Q. *Can my cancer be cured (I am more interested in survival than my sex life)?*

A. As a rough estimate, all patients who have PSAs less than 10, and have early prostate cancer with a Gleason sum score less than 7, have at better than 50% chance of being alive and well 10 years later. This percentage is probably also the case for patients having radical radiotherapy or surgery.

Q. *If it is not curable, can it be controlled?*

A. Hormonal treatment is capable of keeping early disease at bay for many years. Occasionally, radical treatment can be combined with hormonal treatment and once again this can control the disease for many years.

Q. *Do I actually need treatment (cancer confined to prostate gland)?*

A. This is something that you should discuss in detail with your urologist or oncologist. No reputable surgeon or oncologist would mind if you asked for a second opinion. In America, it is not uncommon for patients to have two, three, or even four opinions before opting for treatment.

The Internet can be a great source of information, but do remember that the Internet is not quality controlled and that some of the information is not without bias.

Q. *Why do doctors disagree about what is best (three doctors, three treatments)?*

A. The real reason for this is that there have been no randomized control trials in early prostate cancer. All the evidence that is used is circumstantial. If your doctor is being honest with you, he will find it fairly perplexing and even asking the question 'What would you have done yourself doctor?' would not necessarily meet with a realistic answer. Your doctor has almost certainly not been diagnosed with prostate cancer himself and none of us can really know what this is like, until we have been diagnosed.

Q. *Watchful waiting seems like neglect. What can I do for myself (diet, sex)?*

A. It is probably fair to say that there is very little you can do, other than lead as normal a life as you can and try to forget about your diagnosis as much as possible. Life is for enjoying – it is important that you continue with all your normal activities, including sexual intercourse, if you are able. There is no evidence that altering diet improves survival and you should eat what you feel is best for you.

Q. *What are the disadvantages of watchful waiting?*

A. The main argument here is that the genie can escape from the bottle, in other words, that cancer cells, untreated, can spread from the prostate gland. With careful watchful waiting and surveillance of PSA, there is no evidence that your chances of survival are impaired.

Q. *How often should I be seen by my specialist?*

A. This is best determined in consultation with your urologist, oncologist, or GP; 3–6-monthly seems appropriate in most cases.

Q. *What are the treatment options if a 'wait and see' approach culminates in the progression of prostate cancer?*

A. Assuming that the cancer has not become more advanced, the options are the same as early treatment, mainly radical prostatectomy, radical radiotherapy, or brachytherapy.

Q. *If I wait, will it be more difficult to treat in the future and how fast will it spread?*

A. Assuming you have been under proper surveillance, it is unlikely that the disease will advance to such a state that it becomes untreatable. It is important that you ensure that you and your medical adviser are speaking about the same things.

Unfortunately it is unlikely that we can tell with any accuracy how fast the cancer will spread (the pussycat and tiger story).

Q. *If I have treatment, should this be with surgery or radiotherapy?*

A. This is a matter for discussion and debate. There are advantages and disadvantages with both forms of treatment. Unfortunately, there is no firm evidence that one is 'better' than the other, provided treatment is of the highest quality. The choice is often determined by the balance of the possible side effects (*see* Chapter 4).

Q. *What are the possible adverse side-effects of radical prostatectomy?*

A. As has been discussed earlier, these are of incontinence, impotence, blood loss and death.

Q. *Who would you choose to do your operation?*

A. It makes sense to choose a surgeon who is experienced and can tell you what his particular incontinence and impotence rate is.

Q. *What are the early (temporary) side-effects of radiotherapy?*

A. These include disturbance of bladder function, diarrhoea, and mucus production from the rectum.

Q. *What are the late (permanent) side-effects of radiotherapy?*

A. These are similar to the temporary effects but they are permanent.

Q. *What are the roles of hormone therapy?*

A. Hormone therapy is an excellent way of reducing the effect of the male sex hormone, testosterone, on all forms of prostate tissue, including prostate cancer. In most cases, this does not result in a cure, but rather defers and holds off the disease, usually for about 2 years, but sometimes much longer.

Many thousands of patients have been entered into studies to try and determine this. The idea is that maximum androgen blockade not only interferes with testicular hormones, but also deals with testosterone produced by the adrenal gland. Studies suggest, however, that the benefits of maximum androgen blockade are small or marginal, and it is not routinely used in the UK.

Q. *How can the side-effects of treatment be minimized?*

A. One side-effect that can be quite tedious is that of hot flushes (called this in the UK, hot flashes in the USA). These are usually abolished by using a small 50 mg dosage daily of cyproterone acetate (Cyprostat, Androcur).

Bicalutamide (Casodex) has a major side-effect, in that it causes enlargement of the male breasts, which can be painful. In some cases, oncologists may offer you a small dose of radiotherapy to each breast prior to starting this.

Q. *What about my sex life?*

A. Impotence is a problem for almost all of the treatments. It is less of a problem with bicalutamide and flutamide. Your doctor should discuss with you the importance of sexual function. Do not be shy. It is also important that this is not age related and is a subject which you should expect your doctor to mention.

Q. *How long after my treatment will you be able to tell if my cancer is cured?*

A. There is no effective evidence of cure. What we can say, however, is that the PSA levels taken after radical surgery would be a very good indication as to the degree of prostate activity left. After radical prostatectomy, the PSA level should be virtually unreadable, i.e. less than 0.1 ng/ml.

With radiotherapy, the PSA levels tend to be a bit higher, but it is now accepted at less than 1 or preferably less than 0.5 ng/ml. It is tantamount to a cure. PSA levels can, however, come back and it is at this stage, should this happen, that hormone therapy might be used.

Q. *Why are there not better second-line treatments?*

A.   The level of investment in research in prostate cancer has until recently been very poor. A great deal more money has to be spent if we are even to reach a par with the amount of research that is being pursued, quite rightly, in breast cancer. For too long the disease has been considered one of old men and the fact that many patients are fit and still have the disease has been neglected until recently.

Glossary

Adenocarcinoma   Cancer that appears in glandular tissue such as the prostate.

Adjuvant therapy   Treatment given in addition to the primary therapy.

Adrenal androgen   A male hormone produced by the adrenal glands; adrenal androgens account for about 5 per cent of the body's androgens.

Advanced prostate cancer   Describes the condition where the initial cancer has escaped from the prostate gland to other tissues such as bones and internal organs.

Androgen   Male hormone such as testosterone.

Androgen blockade   Use of drugs to interrupt the activity of male hormones.

Anti-androgen   A drug (usually tablet form) which competes with testosterone and prevents it from functioning.

Benign   Describes a tumour that does not invade and destroy the surrounding tissue or migrate to other sites in the body (compare with malignant) and is therefore not cancerous.

Benign prostatic hyperplasia (BPH)   A non-malignant enlargement of the prostate which can occur with age.

Biopsy   A sample of tissue taken from part of the body (i.e. the prostate gland) which is then analysed under a microscope. A biopsy is normally taken using a small hollow needle.

Bladder neck   Thickened muscle where the bladder joins the urethra. On signal from the brain, this muscle can either tighten or relax to control flow of urine from the bladder to the urethra.

Bladder neck contracture A complication of surgery that causes scarring of the tissue and possible urinary problems. Could require additional surgery to correct.

Bone scan A small, harmless amount of radioactive chemical is injected into the body and is taken-up by the bones. An image can then be created with cancerous tissue showing up as black spots ('hotspots') on the x-ray film. However, not all hotspots are caused by cancer and you may find some old breaks or previous injuries showing up.

Brachytherapy The implantation of radioactive seeds into the prostate gland. These seeds remain in the prostate and give a continual low dose of radiation to the cancerous cells.

Cancer The abnormal and uncontrolled division of cells which may go on to invade and destroy surrounding tissues (see malignant).

Castration The removal of male hormones either through surgical removal of the testicles or with drugs that inhibit hormone production.

Catheter A tube inserted into a narrow opening or orifice (i.e. in the penis) which allows the release of fluids such as urine.

Chemotherapy The treatment or prevention of disease by the use of chemicals. This term is often used to describe anti-cancer drugs which operate by killing rapidly dividing cells.

Cryosurgery The use of freezing liquids to destroy the prostate gland and eliminate the cancer within it.

CT scan Also CAT; computerized axial tomography. A cross-sectional x-ray used in diagnosis and radiation treatment planning.

Cystitis Infection and inflammation of the bladder, which is a possible short-lived side-effect of radiation therapy. Causes painful urination.

DES Diethylstilboestrol, a synthetic oestrogen, used in treatment of prostate cancer.

Differentiated The resemblance of cancer cells to normal cells. Well-differentiated tumour cells closely resemble normal cells and are, therefore, believed to be less aggressive.

Digital rectal examination (DRE) A simple examination carried out by a doctor or nurse where a gloved finger is placed into the patient's back passage where the prostate gland can be felt for abnormalities.

Dysplasia   Abnormal growth of cells.

Dysuria   Burning sensation when urinating.

External beam radiotherapy (EBRT)   The use of high energy x-ray beams which can be used to target and destroy the cells within the prostate gland and surrounding area.

Flutamide   Eulexin, an anti-androgen used in hormonal treatment.

Frequency   The constant need to pass urine, especially at night.

Frozen section   A small piece of a larger piece of tissue taken out during a biopsy that is flash frozen for instant analysis by a pathologist using a microscope to determine whether cancer is present.

FSH   Follicle-stimulating hormone produced by the pituitary gland to activate sperm-forming tubules in the testicles.

Genes (genetics)   All the body's genetic material is in the form of DNA. Lengths of DNA which have a common function, and which code for a particular protein are called genes. When genes become mutated, the resulting proteins are also mutated and may lose their function.

Gene therapy   The use of genetic material to prevent or treat disease. This can include introducing genes into cells which cause the destruction of the cell, or introducing genes which activate other cells to kill the cancer.

Gland   An organ or group of cells which is specialized for the production of fluids such as semen.

Gleason grade   When a biopsy of the prostate is analysed under a microscope, the cells which make up the gland can be examined as to whether they are cancerous, based on their size, shape, and structure. A grade can be supplied to the cells (ranging from 1 to 5) which represents how aggressive the cancer may be (see Table 2.1).

Gleason score   Two Gleason grades are added together from the two representative parts of the biopsy to give a score, i.e. 2 + 4 = score 6 (out of a possible 10).

Goserelin   Zoladex, a synthetic LH-RH agonist/antagonist used in hormonal treatment.

Gray A unit of measure for radiation treatment. Abbreviated as Gy.

Haematuria Blood in the urine.

Hesitancy The need to hesitate before passing urine even when the bladder is full.

Hormone refractory stage A state where prostate cancer cells no longer require testosterone to grow and therefore grow in its absence. Hormone therapy is no longer effective at this point.

Hormone therapy This can be surgical (where the testicles are removed) or medical (where drugs are given). Both procedures lower the ability of testosterone to feed the cancer.

Hormones Substances which are produced in one part of the body and are carried by the blood to another part where they modify the function or structure of other tissues.

Hot flushes These are flushing and a feeling of temperature change associated with facial flushing.

Hyperplasia Abnormal growth of cells due to rapid cell multiplication.

Impotence The inability to achieve an erection firm enough for intercourse to take place.

Incontinence Urinary incontinence is the uncontrolled release of urine from the bladder. This usually involves the constant dribbling of urine and sometimes requires that an incontinence pad or sheath be worn in the underwear.

LH-RH agonist A drug (usually injected into the abdomen) which causes a reduction in testosterone production.

Libido Sexual drive or sexual desire. This can be affected by treatments which alter testosterone function such as medical hormone therapy or orchidectomy.

Localized prostate cancer A condition where the cancerous tissue is contained within the prostate gland (compare with advanced prostate cancer).

Luteinizing hormone (LH) This hormone is secreted by the pituitary gland. It stimulates secretion of androgen by the testicles.

Luteinizing hormone-releasing hormone (LH-RH) This hormone is secreted by the brain to stimulate the secretion of LH by the pituitary gland.

Lymph nodes   Small, bean-shaped organs located along the lumphatic system. Nodes filter bacteria or cancer cells that may travel through the lymphatic system. Also called lymph glands.

Lymphatic system   The tissues and organs, including the bone marrow, spleen, thymus and lymph nodes, that produce and store cells that fight infection and disease.

MAB   Maximal androgen blockade. Hormonal therapy using drugs to completely block the production and activity of male hormones.

Malignant   Describes a tumour which has the ability to destroy tissue or spread to distant sites in the body (compare with benign).

Metastases   Secondary tumours that have migrated from the prostate gland and become established in other sites in the body.

Nocturia   The need to get up frequently at night to urinate.

Oncologist   A doctor who specializes in the treatment of cancer.

Orchidectomy   An operation in which both testicles, or part of both testicles, are removed in order to prevent production of testosterone.

Palliative   Treatment that relieves symptoms such as pain but does not cure.

PIN   Prostatic intraepithelial neoplasia. Believed by some pathologists to be a premalignant lesion if it is high grade.

Priapism   The presence of an erection persisting for more than 4 hours. Medical attention should be sought if this occurs.

Proctitis   Irritation and pain in the rectum and anus, causing diarrhoea and bleeding, a potential side-effect of radiation therapy.

Prostate gland   A gland that is located beneath the bladder and produces secretions which nourish and protect sperm when ejaculated.

Prostatitis   Inflammation of the prostate gland which may be caused by bacterial infection and may respond to antibiotics.

Proteins   The building blocks of life. Proteins are made up of amino acids which are pieced together using genes as a template. Proteins form the structural material that makes up the tissues, organs and muscles as well as forming hormones and other regulatory molecules.

PSA (prostate-specific antigen) A protein found in men which is exclusively produced by the prostate gland. This protein leaks out into the blood where it can be measured.

PSA tests A measurement of PSA in the blood. This level rises when there is a problem with the prostate gland but the test does not differentiate between cancer and other non-malignant conditions.

Radical prostatectomy The complete removal of the prostate gland (compare with TURP).

Radiotherapist A doctor who specializes in radiotherapy in the treatment of disease.

Radiotherapy The use of radiation in the treatment of disease. This radiation can be applied from outside the body (see External Beam Radiotherapy) or from within the body (see brachytherapy).

Seminal vesicles Two glands, like small bunches of grapes, at the top of the prostate and behind the bladder, which produce the sticky substance in semen.

Staging The process carried out to detect whether a cancer is confined or has spread.

Surgeon A doctor who specializes in carrying out operations. This will usually be a urologist who deals with prostate surgery.

Testosterone A male hormone, which is produced mainly by the testicles and is often responsible for feeding prostate cancer and making it grow.

TRUS Transrectal ultrasound scan. The use of an ultrasound probe (similar to that used in the imaging of unborn babies), which is placed inside the back passage and provides an image of the prostate gland. Often used to guide the needle used for biopsy.

Tumour An abnormal growth of tissue which may be benign or malignant.

TURP Transurethral resection of the prostate. The removal of part of the prostate gland from within the penis. The surgical tool, a resectoscope, is placed inside the penis, down the urethra, where the prostate gland is shaved away from the inside.

Urethra The tube which carries urine from the bladder to the opening of the penis. This tube is surrounded by the prostate gland just below the bladder.

Urologist   A doctor who specializes in the treatment of urinary tract diseases such as those affecting the bladder, prostate, and the tubes which carry urine from the kidneys to the bladder.

Vas deferens   Tube through which sperm travels from each testicle to the centre of the prostate in the urethra.

Watchful waiting   The process of observing the patient, giving regular PSA tests, but not actively treating the patient until his symptoms become apparent and require treatment. This form of treatment is valid for many men, who never require radical treatment because they have very slow-growing tumours.

Sources of information

Useful books

Baggish, J. (1995) *Making the Prostate Therapy Decision* (American). Lowell House. ISBN 1–5656520–7X

Haig, S. (ed.) (1995) *Understanding Cancer of the Prostate*. London: British Association of Cancer United Patients (CancerBACUP). ISBN 1–870403–71–1 Available free from BACUP [Tel: (0)20–7696–9003]

Kirk, D. (1995) *Understanding Prostate Disorders* (Family Doctor Series). London: British Medical Association (BMA). ISBN 1–898205–14–0 £2.49

Korda, M. (1997) *Man to Man* (American). Boston: Little Brown. ISBN 0–316–88297–6 £16.99

Loo, M. H. and Betancourt, M. (1998) *The Prostate Cancer Sourcebook*. Chichester: John Wiley & Sons, Inc. ISBN 0–471–15927–1 £11.99

Meyer, S. and Nash, S. (1994) *Prostate Cancer – Making Survival Decisions* (American). Chicago: University of Chicago Press. ISBN 0–226–56857–1 £15.95

Newton, A. C. (1996) *Living with Prostate Cancer*. Toronto: McClelland & Stewart Inc. ISBN 0–7710–6779–8 £8.99

Phillips, R. H. (1994) *Coping with Prostate Cancer*. New York: Avery Publishing Group. ISBN 0–89529–564–4 £9.99

Smith, J. and Gillatt, D. (1996) *Prostate Problems*. London: Hodder & Stoughton. ISBN 0–340–67907–7 £5.99

Useful addresses

The Prostate Cancer Charity
3 Angel Walk, Hammersmith
London W6 9HX
Tel: 020 8383 8124 (general enquiries and donations)
Fax: 020 8383 8126
Helpline: 0845 300 8383
E-mail: info@prostate-cancer.org.uk
Website: *www.prostate-cancer.org.uk*

CancerBACUP (British Association of Cancer United Patients)
3 Bath Place
Rivington Street
London EC2A 3JR
Tel: 020 7696 9003
Fax: 020 7696 9002
Helpline: 020 7613 2121 (from within London)
Freephone: 0800 18 11 99 (from outside London)
Website: *www.bacup.org.uk*

Cancerlink
11–21 Northdown Street
London N1 9BN
Tel: 020 7833 2818 (Administration)
Fax: 020 7833 4963
Helpline: 0808 808 0000
Website: *cancerlink@cancerlink.org.uk*

The Impotence Association
PO Box 10296
London SW17 9WH
Helpline: 020 8767 7791
Website: *www.impotence.org.uk*

The Continence Foundation
307 Hatton Square
16 Baldwins Gardens
London EC1N 7RJ
Tel: 020 7404 6875
Fax: 020 7474 6876
Helpline: 020 7831 9831
Website: *www.vois.org.uk/cf*

Cancer Research UK
PO Box 123
Lincoln's Inn Fields
London WC2A 3PX
Tel: 020 7242 0200
Fax: 020 7269 3101
Website: *www.icnet.uk*

Tenovus Cancer Information Centre
College Buildings
Courtenay Road
Splott
Cardiff CF2 2JP
Helpline: 0808 808 1010
Website: *www.tenovus.org.uk*

Macmillan Cancer Relief
Anchor House
15–19 Britten Street
London SW3 3TZ
Tel: 020 7351 7811
Fax: 020 7376 8098
Helpline: 0845 601 6161
Website: *www.macmillan.org.uk*

The Prostate Health Council
American Federation of Urologic Disease (AFUD)
300 West Pratt Street, Suite 401
Baltimore
MD 21201
Information: 1–800–242–2383
Support Group Network: 1–800–7866

Patient information

Information booklets by CancerBACUP

Coping at Home
Coping with Hair Loss
Facing the Challenge of Advanced Cancer
Feeling Better
Controlling Pain and other Symptoms of Cancer
Understanding Chemotherapy

Understanding Cancer of the Prostate
Understanding Clinical Trials
Understanding Radiotherapy

Other patient publications

The Cancer Guide. Macmillan Cancer Relief.
Bereavement. Help the Aged, St James Walk, Clerkenwell Green,
London EC1R 0BE.

Useful Websites

American Cancer Society: http://www.cancer.org
American Urological Association: http://www.auanet.org
Bacup: http://www.cancerbacup.org.uk
Cancer Research Campaign: http://www.crc.org.uk
CaP CURE: http://www.capcure.org
Guide to Internet resources for cancer: http://www.ncl.ac.uk/child-
health/guides/clinks1.html
National Cancer Institute, USA: http://www.nci.nih.gov
SEER Cancer Statistics: http://www.seer.ims.nci.nih.gov
SIECUS: http://www.siecus.org
Us Too! International: http://www.ustoo.com

Index

Index

Index